THE HEALTHY *heart* HANDBOOK FOR WOMEN

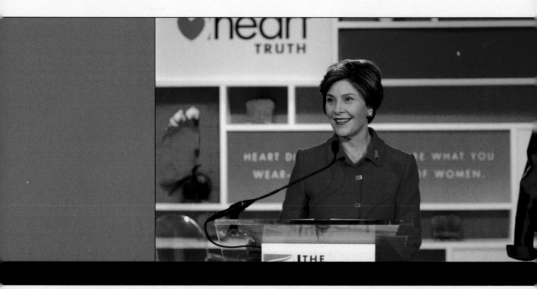

Mrs. Laura Bush, National Ambassador for *The Heart Truth*

Dear Friend,

I applaud you for taking the opportunity to learn more about women and heart disease. *The Healthy Heart Handbook for Women,* written and produced by the experts at the National Heart, Lung, and Blood Institute of the National Institutes of Health as part of its *The Heart Truth* campaign, offers the most up-to-date information on women's heart disease and practical strategies for how to reduce your risk.

Like many women, I had always assumed that heart disease affects mostly men. Yet heart disease is the #1 killer of women in the United States, killing more women than all forms of cancer combined. But the good news is that education, prevention, and even a little red dress can save women's lives.

Thanks to *The Heart Truth,* the red dress has become the national symbol of women's heart health. Women all across the country are taking the message to heart, wearing *The Heart Truth* Red Dress pins, sharing the message with friends and family, and talking to their doctors about their personal risk for heart disease.

I am encouraged by the progress we are making in increasing awareness of women's heart disease, and I urge you to share the information that you learn in this easy-to-use handbook and help spread *The Heart Truth.*

With best wishes,

Laura Bush

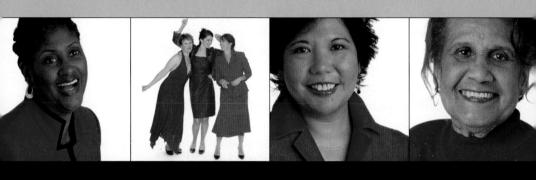

Written by: Marian Sandmaier

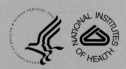

U.S. Department of Health and Human Services
National Institutes of Health

NIH Publication No. 08-2720
Originally printed 1987
Previously revised 1992, 1997, 2003, 2005, 2007
Revised February 2008
Reprinted May 2010

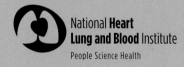

National **Heart**
Lung and Blood Institute
People Science Health

TABLE OF *contents*

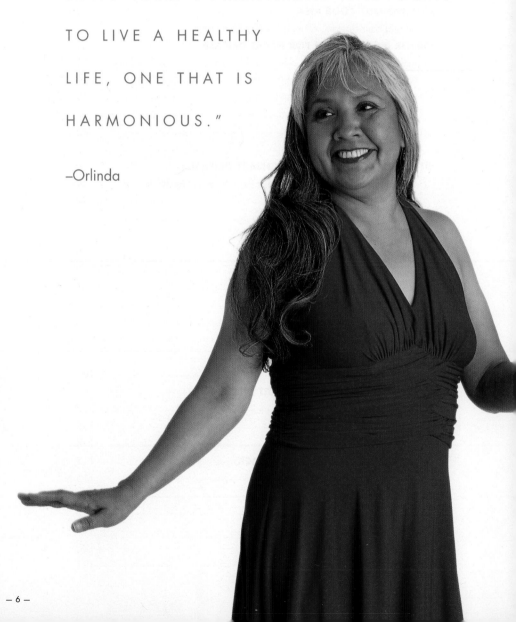

"*THE HEART TRUTH* MEANS TAKING CARE OF YOURSELF AND YOUR HEART—INSIDE AND OUT. IT IS A LONG-TERM COMMITMENT AND GOAL TO LIVE A HEALTHY LIFE, ONE THAT IS HARMONIOUS."

–Orlinda

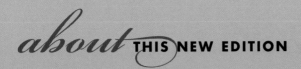

about THIS NEW EDITION

Research on women's heart health is exploding. Nearly every week, it seems, the media report on new ways to prevent and treat heart disease in women—and it can be hard to keep track of it all. In this updated edition of "The Healthy Heart Handbook for Women," we have put together all of this new knowledge in one easy-to-use handbook. This guide is part of *The Heart Truth*, a national public awareness campaign for women about heart disease sponsored by the National Heart, Lung, and Blood Institute (NHLBI) and many other groups. (See "Getting the Word Out" on page 10.)

"The Healthy Heart Handbook for Women" will give you new information on women's heart disease and practical suggestions for reducing your own personal risk of heart-related problems. You'll find out about a little-known form of heart disease in women and how to get it diagnosed properly. The handbook will also help you make sense of widely publicized research on the impact of a lower fat diet on women's heart disease risk.

There is much good news in these pages, including new findings that people who avoid heart disease risk factors tend to live healthier and longer lives. The handbook will give you the latest information on preventing and controlling those risks. You'll also find new tips on following a nutritious eating plan, tailoring your physical activity program to your particular goals, and getting your whole family involved in heart healthy living. The handbook will also advise you on the warning signs of heart attack, as well as how to act quickly to get help.

So welcome to "The Healthy Heart Handbook for Women"—your one-stop source for the latest information on women's heart disease and heart health.

THE *heart* TRUTH

*W*hen you hear the term "heart disease," what is your first reaction? Like many women, you may think, "That's a man's disease" or "Not my problem." But here is *The Heart Truth*: Heart disease is the #1 killer of women in the United States. Most women don't know this. But it is vital that you know it—and know what it means for you.

Some surprising facts:

- One in 4 women in the United States dies of heart disease, while 1 in 30 dies of breast cancer.

- Twenty-three percent of women will die within 1 year after having a heart attack.

- Within 6 years of having a heart attack, about 46 percent of women become disabled with heart failure. Two-thirds of women who have a heart attack fail to make a full recovery.

The fact is, if you've got a heart, heart disease could be your problem. Fortunately, it's a problem you can do something about. This handbook will help you find out your own risk of heart disease and take steps to prevent and control it.

For women in midlife, taking action is particularly important. Once a woman reaches menopause, her risks of heart disease and heart attack jump dramatically. One in eight women between the ages of 45 and 64 has some form of heart disease, and this increases to one in four women over 65.

One in 4 women in the United States dies of heart disease, while 1 in 30 dies of breast cancer.

You still may be thinking, "But this isn't about me. I don't have heart disease." But you may have conditions or habits that can lead to heart disease, such as being overweight, smoking cigarettes, or not engaging in enough physical activity. You may already know about these and other "risk factors" for heart disease. You may know which ones you personally have. What you may not know, though, is that if you have even one risk factor, you are much more likely to develop heart disease, with its many serious consequences. A damaged heart can damage your life by interfering with enjoyable activities and even your ability to do simple things, such as taking a walk or climbing steps.

But now here's the good news: You have tremendous power to prevent heart disease—and you can start today. By learning about your own personal risk factors and by making healthful changes in your diet, physical activity, and other daily habits, you can greatly reduce your risk of developing heart-related problems. Even if you already have heart disease, you can take steps to lessen its severity.

So use this handbook to learn more about heart healthy living. Talk with your physician to get more answers. Start taking action today to protect your heart. As one woman doctor put it, "Heart disease is a 'now' problem. Later may be too late."

GETTING THE *word* OUT

Chances are, you've been seeing and hearing a lot of information lately on women and heart disease. That's because an exciting public awareness campaign is underway to help women protect their heart health. The purpose of this nationwide campaign, called *The Heart Truth*, is to spread the word that heart disease is a women's issue.

The Heart Truth warns women about heart disease and encourages them to take action against its risk factors. The message is paired with an arresting image—the Red Dress—the national symbol for women and heart disease awareness. The symbol links a woman's focus on her "outer self" to the need to also focus on her "inner self," especially her heart health. The Red Dress is a visual "red alert" to convey the message that "Heart Disease Doesn't Care What You Wear—It's the #1 Killer of Women."

The Heart Truth campaign is sponsored by the National Heart, Lung, and Blood Institute in partnership with many national and community health organizations around the country. So the next time you come across a red dress, or a newspaper article or local speaker on women and heart disease, take the time to get the message. *The Heart Truth*: It could save your life.

For more information, visit the campaign's Web pages at **www.hearttruth.gov.**

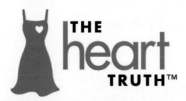

THE **heart** TRUTH™

WHAT IS 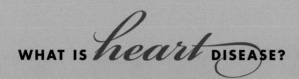DISEASE?

Coronary heart disease—often simply called heart disease—occurs when the arteries that supply blood to the heart muscle become hardened and narrowed due to a buildup of plaque on the arteries' inner walls. Plaque is the accumulation of fat, cholesterol, and other substances. As plaque continues to build up in the arteries, blood flow to the heart is reduced.

Heart disease can lead to a heart attack. A heart attack happens when an artery becomes totally blocked with plaque, preventing vital oxygen and nutrients from getting to the heart. A heart attack can cause permanent damage to the heart muscle.

Heart disease is one of several cardiovascular diseases, which are diseases of the heart and blood vessel system. Other cardiovascular diseases include stroke, high blood pressure, and rheumatic heart disease.

One reason some women aren't too concerned about heart disease is that they think it can be "cured" with surgery. This is a myth. Heart disease is a lifelong condition—once you get it, you'll always have it. True, procedures such as bypass surgery and angioplasty can help blood and oxygen flow to the heart more easily. But the arteries remain damaged, which means you are more likely to have a heart attack.

What's more, the condition of your blood vessels will steadily worsen unless you make changes in your daily habits. Many women die of complications from heart disease or become permanently disabled. That's why it is so vital to take action to prevent and control this disease.

women AT RISK

Risk factors are conditions or habits that make a person more likely to develop a disease. They also can increase the chances that an existing disease will get worse. Important risk factors for heart disease that you can do something about are cigarette smoking, high blood pressure, high blood cholesterol, overweight, physical inactivity, and diabetes. Research shows that more than 95 percent of those who die from heart disease have at least one of these major risk factors.

Some risk factors, such as age and family history of early heart disease, can't be changed. For women, age becomes a risk factor at 55. Women who have gone through early menopause, either naturally or because they have had a hysterectomy, are twice as likely to develop heart disease as women of the same age who have not yet gone through menopause. Another reason for the increasing risk is that middle age is a time when women tend to develop other risk factors for heart disease.

Family history of early heart disease is another risk factor that can't be changed. If your father or brother had a heart attack before age 55, or if your mother or sister had one before age 65, you are more likely to get heart disease yourself.

While certain risk factors cannot be changed, it is important to realize that you do have control over many others. Regardless of your age, background, or health status, you can lower your risk of heart disease—and it doesn't have to be complicated. Protecting your heart can be as simple as taking a brisk walk, whipping up a good vegetable soup, or getting the support you need to maintain a healthy weight.

Every Risk Factor Counts

Some women believe that doing just one healthy thing will take care of all of their heart disease risk. For example, they may think that if they walk or swim regularly, they can still smoke and stay fairly healthy. Wrong! To protect your heart, it is vital to make changes that address each risk factor you have. You can make the changes gradually, one at a time. But making them is very important.

Other women may wonder, "If I have just one risk factor for heart disease—say, I'm overweight or I have high blood cholesterol—aren't I more or less 'safe'?" Absolutely not. Having just one risk factor can double a woman's chance of developing heart disease.

The "Multiplier Effect"

But having more than one risk factor is especially serious, because risk factors tend to "gang up" and worsen each other's effects. Having two risk factors increases the chance of developing heart disease fourfold. Having three or more risk factors increases the chance more than tenfold.

The fact is, most women in midlife already have heart disease risk factors. Thirty-three percent of women ages 40 to 60 have one risk factor for heart disease that they can change. Another 31 percent of women in midlife have two modifiable risk factors, while 17 percent have three or more modifiable risk factors.

Women of color have higher rates of some risk factors. More than 85 percent of African American women in midlife are overweight or obese, while 52 percent have high blood pressure, and 14 percent have been diagnosed with diabetes. Among Hispanic women in midlife, 78 percent are overweight or obese, while more than 10 percent have been diagnosed with diabetes.

The message is clear: Every woman needs to take her heart disease risk seriously—and take action now to reduce that risk.

DID *you* KNOW?

Many women think that breast cancer is a bigger threat than heart disease. But the leading causes of death for American women in the year 2004* were:

Heart Disease _____ 332,313

Cancer (all types) _____ 265,022

- Lung _____ 67,838
- Breast _____ 40,539
- Colorectal _____ 26,762
- Pancreatic _____ 15,815
- Ovarian _____ 14,593
- Uterine _____ 6,906
- Cervical _____ 3,804
- Others _____ 88,765

Stroke _____ 91,487

Chronic Obstructive Pulmonary Disease _____ 64,409

Alzheimer's Disease _____ 46,954

Accidents _____ 38,903

Diabetes _____ 37,771

Pneumonia/Influenza _____ 33,902

* Most recent year for which data are available.

FINDING OUT *your* RISK

The first step toward heart health is becoming aware of your own personal risk for heart disease. Some risks, such as smoking cigarettes, are obvious: Every woman knows whether or not she smokes. But other risk factors, such as high blood pressure or high blood cholesterol, generally don't have obvious signs or symptoms. So you'll need to gather some information to create your personal "heart profile."

You and Your Doctor: A Heart Healthy Partnership

A crucial step in determining your risk is to see your doctor for a thorough checkup. Your physician can be an important partner in helping you set and reach goals for heart health. But don't wait for your doctor to mention heart disease or its risk factors. Many doctors don't routinely bring up the subject with women patients. Research shows that women are less likely than men to receive heart healthy recommendations from their doctors. Here are some tips for establishing good, clear communication between you and your doctor:

Speak up. Tell your doctor you want to keep your heart healthy and would like help in achieving that goal. Ask questions about your chances of developing heart disease and how you can lower your risk. (See "Questions To Ask Your Doctor" on page 17.) Also ask for tests that will determine your personal risk factors. (See "Check It Out" on pages 18 and 19.)

Keep tabs on treatment. If you already are being treated for heart disease or heart disease risk factors, ask your doctor to review your treatment plan with you. Ask, "Is what I'm doing in line with the latest recommendations? Are my treatments working? Are my risk factors under control?" If your doctor recommends a medical procedure, ask about its benefits and risks. Find out if you will need to be hospitalized and for how long, and what to expect during the recovery period.

Be open. When your doctor asks you questions, answer as honestly and fully as you can. While certain topics may seem quite personal, discussing them openly can help your doctor find out your chances of developing heart disease. It can also help your doctor work with you to reduce your risk. If you already have heart disease, briefly describe each of your symptoms. Include when each symptom started, how often it happens, and whether it has been getting worse.

Keep it simple. If you don't understand something your doctor says, ask for an explanation in simple language. Be especially sure you understand how to take any medication you are given. If you are worried about understanding what the doctor says, or if you have trouble hearing, bring a friend or relative with you to your appointment. You may want to ask that person to write down the doctor's instructions for you.

QUESTIONS TO ASK YOUR *doctor*

Getting answers to these questions will give you vital information about your heart health and what you can do to improve it. You may want to take this list to your doctor's office:

1. What is my risk for heart disease?

2. What is my blood pressure? What does it mean for me, and what do I need to do about it?

3. What are my cholesterol numbers? (These include total cholesterol, LDL or "bad" cholesterol, HDL or "good" cholesterol, and triglycerides.) What do they mean for me, and what do I need to do about them?

4. What are my body mass index (BMI) and waist measurement? Do they indicate that I need to lose weight for my health?

5. What is my blood sugar level, and does it mean I'm at risk for diabetes?

6. What other screening tests for heart disease do I need? How often should I return for checkups for my heart health?

7. What can you do to help me quit smoking?

8. How much physical activity do I need to help protect my heart?

9. What is a heart healthy eating plan for me? Should I see a registered dietitian or qualified nutritionist to learn more about healthy eating?

10. How can I tell if I'm having a heart attack?

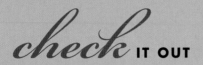 **IT OUT**

Tests That Can Help Protect Your Heart Health
Ask your doctor to give you these tests. Each one will give you valuable information about your heart disease risk.

Lipoprotein Profile
What: A blood test that measures total cholesterol, HDL or "good" cholesterol, LDL or "bad" cholesterol, and triglycerides, another form of fat in the blood. The test is given after a 9- to 12-hour fast.

Why: To find out if you have any of the following: high blood cholesterol (high total and LDL cholesterol), low HDL cholesterol, or high triglyceride levels. All affect your risk for heart disease.

When: All healthy adults should have their blood cholesterol levels checked at least once every 5 years. Depending on the results, your doctor may want to repeat the test more frequently.

Blood Pressure
What: A simple, painless test using an inflatable cuff on the arm.

Why: To find out if you have high blood pressure (also called hypertension) or prehypertension. Both are risk factors for heart disease.

When: At least every 2 years, or more often if you have high blood pressure or prehypertension.

Fasting Plasma Glucose

What: The preferred test for diagnosing diabetes. After you have fasted overnight, you will get a blood test the following morning.

Why: To find out if you have diabetes or are likely to develop the disease. Fasting plasma glucose levels of more than 126 mg/dL on two tests on different days mean that you have diabetes. Levels between 100 and 125 mg/dL mean you have an increased risk for diabetes and may have prediabetes. Diabetes is an important risk factor for heart disease and other medical disorders.

When: At least every 3 years, beginning at age 45. If you have risk factors for diabetes, you should be tested at a younger age and more often.

Body Mass Index (BMI) and Waist Circumference

What: BMI is a measure of your weight in relation to your height. Waist circumference is a measure of the fat around your middle.

Why: To find out whether your body type raises your risk of heart disease. A BMI of 25 or higher means you are overweight. A BMI of 30 or higher means you are obese. Both overweight and obesity are risk factors for heart disease. For women, a waist measurement of more than 35 inches increases the risk of heart disease and other serious health conditions.

When: Every 2 years, or more often if your doctor recommends it.

Other Tests

There also are several tests that can determine whether you already have heart disease. Ask your doctor whether you need a stress test, an electrocardiogram (EKG or ECG), or another diagnostic test. (See "Screening Tests" on page 107.)

WHAT'S *your* RISK?

Here is a quick quiz to find out your risk of a heart attack.

	Yes	No	Don't Know
Do you smoke?			
Is your blood pressure 140/90 mmHg or higher, OR have you been told by your doctor that your blood pressure is too high?			
Has your doctor told you that your LDL ("bad") cholesterol is too high, OR that your total cholesterol level is 200 mg/dL or higher, OR that your HDL ("good") cholesterol is less than 40 mg/dL?			
Has your father or brother had a heart attack before age 55, OR has your mother or sister had one before age 65?			
Do you have diabetes OR a fasting blood sugar of 126 mg/dL or higher, OR do you need medicine to control your blood sugar?			
Are you over 55 years old?			
Do you have a body mass index (BMI) score of 25 or more? (To find out, see page 41.)			
Do you get less than a total of 30 minutes of moderate-intensity physical activity on most days?			
Has a doctor told you that you have angina (chest pains), OR have you had a heart attack?			

If you checked any of the "yes" boxes, you're at an increased risk of having a heart attack. If you checked "don't know" for any questions, ask your doctor for help in answering them. Read on to learn what you can do to lower your risk.

MAJOR RISK FACTORS FOR *heart* DISEASE

*A*s important as it is to work closely with your doctor, it is only the first step. To make a lasting difference in your heart health, you'll also need to educate yourself about heart disease and about the kinds of habits and conditions that can raise your risk. It's your heart, and you're in charge. What follows is a basic guide to the most important risk factors for heart disease and how each of them affects a woman's health.

Smoking

Smoking is "the leading cause of preventable death and disease in the United States," according to the Centers for Disease Control and Prevention. Women who smoke are two to six times more likely to suffer a heart attack than nonsmoking women, and the risk increases with the number of cigarettes smoked each day. Smoking can also shorten a healthy life, because smokers are likely to suffer a heart attack or other major heart problem at least 10 years sooner than nonsmokers. Smoking also raises the risk of stroke.

But heart disease and stroke are not the only health risks for women who smoke. Smoking greatly increases the chances that a woman will develop lung cancer. In fact, the lung cancer death rate for women is now higher than the death rate for breast cancer. Cigarette smoking also causes many other types of cancer, including cancers of the mouth, urinary tract, kidney, and cervix. Smoking also causes most cases of chronic obstructive lung disease, which includes bronchitis and emphysema.

If you smoke indoors, the "secondhand smoke" from your cigarettes can cause heart disease, lung cancer, and other serious health problems in the nonsmokers around you. According to a recent report from the U.S. Surgeon General, exposure to smoke at home or work increases a nonsmoker's risk of developing heart disease by 25 to 30 percent. Secondhand smoke is especially harmful to infants and young children, causing breathing problems, ear infections, asthma attacks, and sudden infant death syndrome (SIDS).

Currently, about 20 percent of American women are smokers. In addition, 26 percent of high school seniors smoke at least one cigarette per month. In young people, smoking can interfere with lung growth and causes more frequent and severe respiratory illnesses, in addition to increasing heart disease and cancer risks. The younger people start smoking, the more likely they are to become strongly addicted to nicotine.

There is simply no safe way to smoke. Low-tar and low-nicotine cigarettes do not lessen the risks of heart disease or other smoking-related diseases. The only safe and healthful course is not to smoke at all. (For tips on how to quit, see "You *Can* Stop Smoking" on page 101.)

High Blood Pressure

High blood pressure, also known as hypertension, is another major risk factor for heart disease, as well as for kidney disease and congestive heart failure. High blood pressure is also the most important risk factor for stroke. Even slightly high levels increase your risk for these conditions.

New research shows that at least 65 million adults in the United States have high blood pressure—a 30-percent increase over the last several years. Equally worrisome, blood pressure levels have increased substantially for American children and teens, raising their risk of developing hypertension in adulthood.

Major contributors to high blood pressure are a family history of the disease, overweight, and eating a diet high in salt and sodium. Older individuals are at higher risk than younger people. Among older individuals, women are more likely than men to develop high blood pressure. African American women are more likely to develop high blood pressure, and at earlier ages, than White women. But nearly all of us are at risk, especially as we grow older. Middle-aged Americans who don't currently have high blood pressure have a 90-percent chance of eventually developing the disease.

High blood pressure is often called the "silent killer," because it usually doesn't cause symptoms. As a result, many people pay little attention to their blood pressure until they become seriously ill. According to a national survey, two-thirds of people with high blood pressure do not have it under control. The good news is that you can take action to control or prevent high blood pressure, and thereby avoid many life-threatening disorders. Another new blood pressure category, called prehypertension, has been created to alert people to their increased risk of developing high blood pressure so that they can take steps to prevent the disease.

What Is Blood Pressure?
Blood pressure is the amount of force exerted by the blood against the walls of the arteries. Everyone has to have some blood pressure so that blood can get to all of the body's organs.

Usually, blood pressure is expressed as two numbers, such as 120/80, and is measured in millimeters of mercury (mmHg). The first number is the systolic blood pressure, the amount of force used when the heart beats. The second number, or diastolic blood pressure, is the pressure that exists in the arteries between heartbeats.

Because blood pressure changes often, your health care provider should check it on several different days before deciding whether your blood pressure is too high. Blood pressure is considered "high" when it stays above prehypertensive levels over a period of time. (See next page.)

Understanding Risk

But numbers don't tell the whole story. For example, if you have prehypertension, you are still at increased risk for a heart attack, stroke, or heart failure. Also, if your systolic blood pressure (first number) is 140 mmHg or higher, you are more likely to develop cardiovascular and kidney diseases even if your diastolic blood pressure (second number) is not too high. Starting around age 55, women are more likely to develop high systolic blood pressure. High systolic blood pressure *is* high blood pressure. If you have this condition, you will need to take steps to control it. High blood pressure can be controlled in two ways: by changing your lifestyle and by taking medication.

BLOOD PRESSURE: HOW *high* IS HIGH?

Your blood pressure is determined by the higher number of either your systolic or your diastolic measurement. For example, if your systolic number is 115 mmHg but your diastolic number is 85 mmHg, your category is prehypertension.

	Systolic	Diastolic
Normal	Less than 120 mmHg	Less than 80 mmHg
Prehypertension	120–139 mmHg	80–89 mmHg
Hypertension	140 mmHg or higher	90 mmHg or higher

Changing Your Lifestyle

If your blood pressure is not too high, you may be able to control it entirely by losing weight if you are overweight, getting regular physical activity, cutting down on alcohol, and changing your eating habits. A special eating plan called "DASH" can help you lower your blood pressure. DASH stands for "Dietary Approaches to Stop Hypertension."

The DASH eating plan emphasizes fruits, vegetables, fat-free or low-fat milk and milk products, whole-grain products, fish, poultry, beans, seeds, and nuts. The DASH eating plan also contains less salt/sodium, sweets, added sugars, sugar containing beverages, fats, and red meats than the typical American diet. This heart healthy way of eating is lower in saturated fat, and cholesterol, and is rich in nutrients that are associated with lowering blood pressure—mainly potassium, magnesium, calcium, protein, and fiber.

If you follow the DASH eating plan and also consume less sodium, you are likely to reduce your blood pressure even more. Sodium is a substance that affects blood pressure and is the main ingredient in salt.

Because fruits and vegetables are naturally lower in sodium than many other foods, DASH makes it easier to eat less sodium. Try it at the 2,300 milligram level (about 1 teaspoon of table salt). Then, talk to your doctor about gradually lowering it to 1,500 milligrams a day. Choose and prepare foods with less salt and don't bring the salt shaker to the table. And remember, salt/sodium is found in many processed foods, such as soups, convenience meals, some breads and cereals, and salted snacks.

For more on the DASH eating plan and how to make other changes that can lower and prevent high blood pressure, see "Taking Control" on page 60 of this handbook.

PREVENTING CONGESTIVE HEART FAILURE

High blood pressure is the #1 risk factor for congestive heart failure. Heart failure is a life-threatening condition in which the heart cannot pump enough blood to supply the body's needs. Congestive heart failure occurs when excess fluid starts to leak into the lungs, causing tiredness, weakness, and breathing difficulties.

To prevent congestive heart failure, and stroke as well, you must control your high blood pressure to below 140/90 mmHg. If your blood pressure is higher than that, talk with your doctor about starting or adjusting medication, as well as making lifestyle changes.

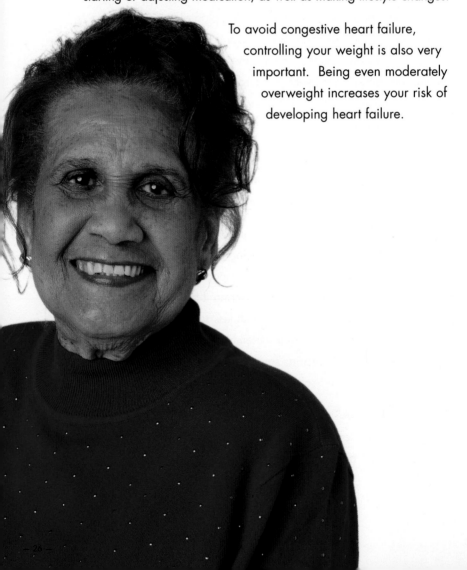

To avoid congestive heart failure, controlling your weight is also very important. Being even moderately overweight increases your risk of developing heart failure.

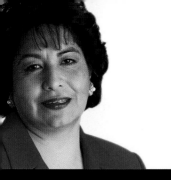

ROSARIO

"I have to lose weight and reduce my cholesterol. This is just the beginning of a long battle, and I know it won't be easy, but I know I have to do it."

Taking Medication

If your blood pressure remains high even after you make lifestyle changes, your doctor will probably prescribe medicine. Lifestyle changes will help the medicine work more effectively. In fact, if you are successful with the changes you make in your daily habits, then you may be able to gradually reduce how much medication you take.

Taking medicine to lower blood pressure can reduce your risk of stroke, heart attack, congestive heart failure, and kidney disease. If you take a drug and notice any uncomfortable side effects, ask your doctor about changing the dosage or switching to another type of medicine.

A recent study found diuretics (water pills) work better than newer drugs to treat hypertension and to prevent some forms of heart disease. If you're starting treatment for high blood pressure, try a diuretic first. If you need more than one drug, ask your doctor about making one a diuretic. And, if you're already taking medicine for high blood pressure, ask about switching to or adding a diuretic. Diuretics work for most people, but if you need a different drug, others are very effective. To make the best choice, talk with your doctor.

Remember, it is important to take blood pressure medication exactly as your doctor has prescribed it. Before you leave your doctor's office, be sure you understand the amount of medicine you are supposed to take each day and the specific times of day you should take it.

STROKE: *know* THE WARNING SIGNS

Stroke is a medical emergency. If you or someone you know has a stroke, it is important to recognize the symptoms so you can get to a hospital quickly. Getting treatment within 60 minutes can prevent disability. The chief warning signs of a stroke are:

- Sudden numbness or weakness of the face, arm, or leg (especially on one side of the body).

- Sudden confusion, trouble speaking, or understanding speech.

- Sudden trouble seeing in one or both eyes.

- Sudden trouble walking, dizziness, or loss of balance or coordination.

- Sudden severe headache with no known cause.

If you think someone might be having a stroke, dial 9–1–1 immediately. Also, be sure that family members and others close to you know the warning signs of a stroke. Give them a copy of this list. Ask them to call 9–1–1 right away if you or someone else shows any signs of a stroke.

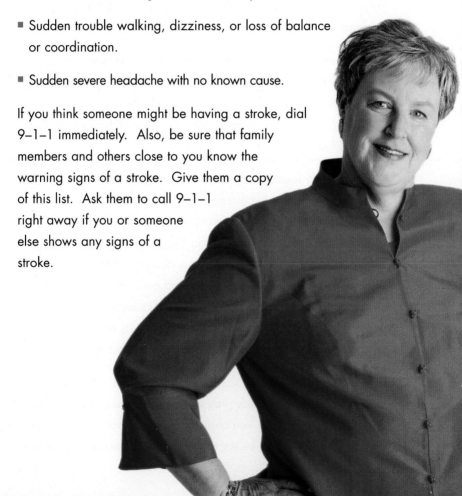

High Blood Cholesterol

High blood cholesterol is another major risk factor for heart disease that you can do something about. The higher your blood cholesterol level, the greater your risk for developing heart disease or having a heart attack. To prevent these disorders, all women should make a serious effort to keep their cholesterol at healthy levels.

If you already have heart disease, it is particularly important to lower an elevated blood cholesterol level to reduce your high risk for a heart attack. Women with diabetes also are at especially high risk for a heart attack. If you have diabetes, you will need to take steps to keep both your cholesterol and your diabetes under control.

Although young women tend to have lower cholesterol levels than young men, between the ages of 45 and 55, women's levels begin to rise higher than men's. After age 55, this "cholesterol gap" between women and men becomes still wider. Although women's overall risk of heart disease at older ages continues to be somewhat lower than that of men, the higher a woman's blood cholesterol level, the greater her chances of developing heart disease.

Cholesterol and Your Heart

The body needs cholesterol to function normally. However, your body makes all the cholesterol it needs. Over a period of years, extra cholesterol and fat circulating in the blood build up in the walls of the arteries that supply blood to the heart. This buildup, called plaque, makes the arteries narrower and narrower. As a result, less blood gets to the heart. Blood carries oxygen to the heart. If not enough oxygen-rich blood can reach your heart, you may suffer chest pain. If the blood supply to a portion of the heart is completely cut off, the result is a heart attack.

Cholesterol travels in the blood in packages called lipoproteins. LDL carries most of the cholesterol in the blood. Cholesterol packaged in LDL is often called "bad" cholesterol, because too much LDL in the blood can lead to cholesterol buildup and blockage in the arteries.

Another type of cholesterol is HDL, known as "good" cholesterol. That's because HDL helps remove cholesterol from the body, preventing it from building up in the arteries.

Getting Tested

High blood cholesterol itself does not cause symptoms, so if your cholesterol level is too high, you may not be aware of it. That's why it's important to get your cholesterol levels checked regularly. Starting at age 20, all women should have their cholesterol levels checked by means of a blood test called a "fasting lipoprotein profile." Be sure to ask for the test results, so you will know whether you need to lower your cholesterol. Ask your doctor how soon you should be retested.

Total cholesterol is a measure of the cholesterol in all of your lipoproteins, including the "bad" cholesterol in LDL and the "good" cholesterol in HDL. An LDL level below 100 mg/dL* is considered "optimal," or ideal. However, not every woman needs to aim for so low a level. As you can see on the next page, there are four other categories of LDL level. The higher your LDL number, the higher your risk of heart disease. Knowing your LDL number is especially important because it will determine the kind of treatment you may need.

Your HDL number tells a different story. The lower your HDL level, the higher your heart disease risk.

Your lipoprotein profile test will also measure levels of triglycerides, another fatty substance in the blood. (See "What Are Triglycerides?" on page 33.)

* Cholesterol levels are measured in milligrams (mg) of cholesterol per deciliter (dL) of blood.

What's Your Number?

Blood Cholesterol Levels and Heart Disease Risk

Total Cholesterol Level	Category
Less than 200 mg/dL	Desirable
200–239 mg/dL	Borderline high
240 mg/dL and above	High

LDL Cholesterol Level	Category
Less than 100 mg/dL	Optimal (ideal)
100–129 mg/dL	Near optimal/above optimal
130–159 mg/dL	Borderline high
160–189 mg/dL	High
190 mg/dL and above	Very high

HDL Cholesterol Level

An HDL cholesterol level of less than 40 mg/dL is a major risk factor for heart disease. An HDL level of 60 mg/dL or higher is somewhat protective.

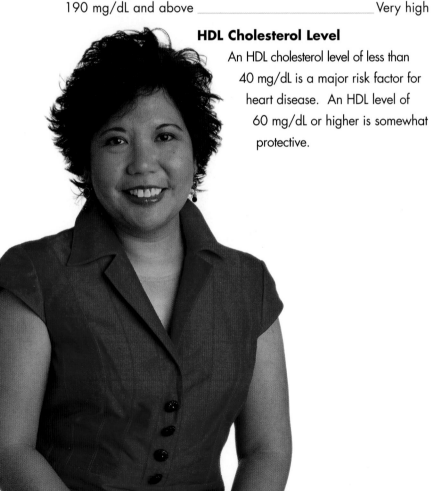

Heart Disease Risk and Your LDL Goal

In general, the higher your LDL level and the more other risk factors you have, the greater your chances of developing heart disease or having a heart attack. The higher your risk, the lower your LDL goal level will be. Here is how to determine your LDL goal:

Step 1: Count your risk factors. Below are risk factors for heart disease that will affect your LDL goal. Check to see how many of the following risk factors* you have:

- Cigarette smoking

- High blood pressure (140/90 mmHg or higher, or if you are on blood pressure medication)

- Low HDL cholesterol (less than 40 mg/dL)[†]

- Family history of early heart disease (your father or brother before age 55, or your mother or sister before age 65)

- Age (55 or older)

Step 2: Find Out Your Risk Score. If you have two or more risk factors in Step 1, you will need to figure out your "risk score." This score will show your chances of having a heart attack in the next 10 years. To find out your risk score, see "How To Estimate Your Risk" on page 120.

---

* Diabetes is not on the list because a person with diabetes is already considered to be at high risk for a heart attack—at the same level of risk as someone who has heart disease. Also, even though overweight and physical inactivity are not on this list of risk factors, they are conditions that raise your risk for heart disease and need to be corrected.

† If your HDL cholesterol is 60 mg/dL or higher, subtract 1 from your total.

Step 3: Find Out Your Risk Category. Use your number of risk factors, risk score, and medical history to find out your category of risk for heart disease or heart attack. Use the table below:

If You Have _____ **Your Category Is**

Heart disease, diabetes, or a
risk score of more than 20 percent _____ High Risk

2 or more risk factors and
a risk score of 10 to 20 percent _____ Next Highest Risk

2 or more risk factors and
a risk score of less than 10 percent _____ Moderate Risk

0 to 1 risk factor _____ Low-to-Moderate Risk

what ARE TRIGLYCERIDES?

Triglycerides are another type of fat found in the blood and in food. Triglycerides are produced in the liver. When you drink alcohol or take in more calories than your body needs, your liver produces more triglycerides. Triglyceride levels that are borderline high (150–199 mg/dL) or high (200–499 mg/dL) are signals of an increased risk for heart disease. To reduce blood triglyceride levels, it is important to control your weight, get more physical activity, quit smoking, and avoid alcohol. You should also follow an eating plan that is not too high in carbohydrates (less than 60 percent of calories) and is low in saturated fat, *trans* fat, and cholesterol. Sometimes, medication is also needed.

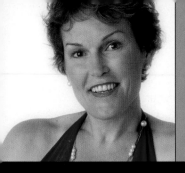

A Special Type of Risk

Some women have a group of risk factors known as "metabolic syndrome," which is usually caused by overweight or obesity and by not getting enough physical activity. This cluster of risk factors increases your risk of heart disease and diabetes, regardless of your LDL cholesterol level. Women have metabolic syndrome if they have three or more of the following conditions:

- A waist measurement of 35 inches or more
- Triglycerides of 150 mg/dL or more
- An HDL level of less than 50 mg/dL
- Blood pressure of 130/85 mmHg or more (either number counts)
- Blood sugar of 100 mg/dL or more

If you have metabolic syndrome, you should calculate your risk score and risk category as indicated in Steps 2 and 3 on the previous page.

You should make a particularly strong effort to reach and maintain your LDL goal. You should emphasize weight control and physical activity to correct the risk factors of the metabolic syndrome.

Your LDL Goal

The main goal of cholesterol-lowering treatment is to lower your
LDL level enough to reduce your risk of heart disease or heart
attack. The higher your risk category, the lower your LDL goal
will be. To find your personal LDL goal, see the table below:

If You Are in This Risk Category	Your LDL Goal Is
High Risk	Less than 100 mg/dL
Next Highest Risk or Moderate Risk	Less than 130 mg/dL
Low-to-Moderate Risk	Less than 160 mg/dL

Recent studies have added to the evidence suggesting that for
people with heart disease, lower LDL cholesterol is better. Because
these studies show a direct relationship between lower LDL
cholesterol and reduced risk for heart attack, it is now reasonable
for doctors to set the LDL treatment goal for heart disease patients at
less than 70 mg/dL—well below the recommended level of less
than 100 mg/dL. Doctors may also use more intensive cholesterol-
lowering treatment to help patients reach this goal.

If you have heart disease, work with your doctor to lower your LDL
cholesterol as much as possible. But even if you can't lower your
LDL cholesterol to less than 70 mg/dL because of a high starting
level, lowering your LDL cholesterol to less than 100 mg/dL will still
greatly reduce your risk.

How To Lower Your LDL

There are two main ways to lower your LDL cholesterol—through lifestyle changes alone, or though medication combined with lifestyle changes. Depending on your risk category, the use of these treatments will differ.

Because of the recent studies that showed the benefit of more intensive cholesterol lowering, physicians have the option to start cholesterol medication—in addition to lifestyle therapy—at lower LDL levels than previously recommended for high-risk patients. For information on the updated treatment options and the best treatment plan for your risk category, see the fact sheet, "High Blood Cholesterol: What You Need To Know," available on the NHLBI Web site or from the NHLBI Health Information Center. (See "To Learn More" on page 121.)

Lifestyle Changes. One important treatment approach is called the TLC Program. TLC stands for "Therapeutic Lifestyle Changes," a three-part treatment that uses diet, physical activity, and weight management. Every woman who needs to lower her LDL cholesterol should use the TLC Program. (For more on the TLC approach, see page 72.) Maintaining a healthy weight and getting regular physical activity are especially important for women who have metabolic syndrome.

Medication. If your LDL level stays too high even after making lifestyle changes, you may need to take medicine. If you need medication, be sure to use it along with the TLC approach. This will keep the dose of medicine as low as possible and lower your risk in other ways as well. You will also need to control all of your other heart disease risk factors, including high blood pressure, diabetes, and smoking.

CHOLESTEROL-LOWERING MEDICINES

As part of your cholesterol-lowering treatment plan, your doctor may recommend medication. The most commonly used medicines are listed below.

Statins. These are the most commonly prescribed drugs for people who need a cholesterol-lowering medicine. They lower LDL levels more than other types of drugs—about 20 to 55 percent. They also moderately lower triglycerides and raise HDL. Side effects are usually mild, although liver and muscle problems may occur rarely. If you experience muscle aches or weakness, you should contact your doctor promptly.

Ezetimibe. This is the first in a new class of cholesterol-lowering drugs that interferes with the absorption of cholesterol in the intestine. Ezetimbe lowers LDL by about 18 to 25 percent. It can be used alone or in combination with a statin to get more lowering of LDL. Side effects may include back and joint pain.

Bile acid resins. These medications lower LDL cholesterol by about 15 to 30 percent. Bile acid resins are often prescribed along with a statin to further decrease LDL cholesterol levels. Side effects may include constipation, bloating, nausea, and gas. However, long-term use of these medicines is considered safe.

Niacin. Niacin, or nicotinic acid, lowers total cholesterol, LDL cholesterol, and triglyceride levels, while also raising HDL cholesterol. It reduces LDL levels by about 5 to 15 percent, and up to 25 percent in some patients. Although niacin is available without a prescription, it is important to use it only under a doctor's care because of possibly serious side effects. In some people, it may worsen peptic ulcers or cause liver problems, gout, or high blood sugar.

Fibrates. These drugs can reduce triglyceride levels by 20 to 50 percent, while increasing HDL cholesterol by 10 to 15 percent. Fibrates are not very effective for lowering LDL cholesterol. The drugs can increase the chances of developing gallstones and heighten the effects of blood-thinning drugs.

Overweight and Obesity

A healthy weight is important for a long, vigorous life. Yet overweight and obesity (extreme overweight) have reached epidemic levels in the United States. About 62 percent of all American women age 20 and older are overweight—about 33 percent of them are obese (extremely overweight). The more overweight a woman is, the higher her risk for heart disease. Overweight also increases the risks for stroke, congestive heart failure, gallbladder disease, arthritis, and breathing problems, as well as for breast, colon, and other cancers.

Overweight in children is also swiftly increasing. Among young people 6 to 19 years old, more than 16 percent are overweight, compared to just 4 percent a few decades ago. This is a disturbing trend because overweight teens have a greatly increased risk of dying from heart disease in adulthood. Even our youngest citizens are at risk. About 10 percent of preschoolers weigh more than is healthy for them.

Our national waistline is expanding for two simple reasons—we are eating more and moving less. Today, Americans consume about 200 to 300 more calories per day than they did in the 1970s. Moreover, as we spend more time in front of computers, video games, TV, and other electronic pastimes, we have fewer hours available for physical activity. There is growing evidence of a link between "couch potato" behavior and an increased risk of obesity and many chronic diseases.

It is hard to overstate the dangers of an unhealthy weight. If you are overweight, you are more likely to develop heart disease even if you have no other risk factors. Overweight and obesity also increase the risks for diabetes, high blood pressure, high blood cholesterol, stroke, congestive heart failure, gallbladder disease, arthritis, breathing problems, and gout, as well as for cancers of the breast and colon.

Each year, an estimated 300,000 U.S. adults die of diseases related to obesity. The bottom line is that maintaining a healthy weight is an extremely important part of heart disease prevention. It can help to protect your health—and may even save your life.

Should You Choose To Lose?

Do you need to lose weight to reduce your risk of heart disease? You can find out by taking three simple steps.

Step 1: Get your number. Take a look at the box on page 41. You'll notice that your weight in relation to your height gives you a number called a "body mass index" (BMI). A BMI of 18.5 to 24.9 indicates a normal weight. A person with a BMI from 25 to 29.9 is overweight, while someone with a BMI of 30 or higher is obese. Those in the "overweight" or "obese" categories have a higher risk of heart disease—and the higher the BMI, the greater the risk.

Step 2: Take out a tape measure. For women, a waist measurement of more than 35 inches increases the risk of heart disease as well as the risks of high blood pressure, diabetes, and other serious health conditions. To measure your waist correctly, stand and place a tape measure around your middle, just above your hip bones. Measure your waist just after you breathe out.

Step 3: Review your risk. The final step in determining your need to lose weight is to find out your other risk factors for heart disease. It is important to know whether you have any of the following: high blood pressure, high LDL cholesterol, low HDL cholesterol, high triglycerides, high blood glucose (blood sugar), physical inactivity, smoking, or a family history of early heart disease. Being age 55 or older or having gone through menopause also increases risk. If you have a condition known as metabolic syndrome (see page 34), your risk of heart disease is particularly high. If you aren't sure whether you have some of these risk factors, ask your doctor.

Once you have taken these three steps, you can use the information to decide whether you need to take off pounds. Although you should talk with your doctor about whether you should lose weight, keep these guidelines in mind:

- If you are overweight AND have two or more other risk factors, or if you are obese, you should lose weight.

- If you are overweight, have a waist measurement of more than 35 inches, AND have two or more other risk factors, you should lose weight.

- If you are overweight, but do not have a high waist measurement and have fewer than two other risk factors, you should avoid further weight gain.

ARE YOU AT A *healthy* WEIGHT?

Body Mass Index

Here is a chart for men and women that gives the BMI for various heights and weights.*

BODY MASS INDEX

HEIGHT	21	22	23	24	25	26	27	28	29	30	31
4'10"	100	105	110	115	119	124	129	134	138	143	148
5'0"	107	112	118	123	128	133	138	143	148	153	158
5'1"	111	116	122	127	132	137	143	148	153	158	164
5'3"	118	124	130	135	141	146	152	158	163	169	175
5'5"	126	132	138	144	150	156	162	168	174	180	186
5'7"	134	140	146	153	159	166	172	178	185	191	198
5'9"	142	149	155	162	169	176	182	189	196	203	209
5'11"	150	157	165	172	179	186	193	200	208	215	222
6'1"	159	166	174	182	189	197	204	212	219	227	235
6'3"	168	176	184	192	200	208	216	224	232	240	248

* Weight is measured with underwear but no shoes.

What Does Your BMI Mean?

Normal weight: BMI = 18.5–24.9. Good for you! Try not to gain weight.

Overweight: BMI = 25–29.9. Do not gain any weight, especially if your waist measurement is high. You need to lose weight if you have two or more risk factors for heart disease and are overweight, or have a high waist measurement.

Obese: BMI = 30 or greater. You need to lose weight. Lose weight slowly— about $1/2$ to 2 pounds a week. See your doctor or a nutritionist if you need help.

Source: "Clinical Guidelines on the Identification, Evaluation, and Treatment of Overweight and Obesity in Adults: The Evidence Report," National Heart, Lung, and Blood Institute, in cooperation with the National Institute of Diabetes and Digestive and Kidney Diseases, National Institutes of Health, NIH Publication 98-4083, June 1998.

Small Changes Make a Big Difference

If you need to lose weight, here is some good news: a small weight loss—just 5 to 10 percent of your current weight—will help to lower your risks of heart disease and other serious medical disorders. The best way to take off pounds is to do so gradually, by getting more physical activity and following a heart healthy eating plan that is lower in calories and fat. (High-fat foods contain more calories than the same amount of other foods, so they can make it hard for you to avoid excess calories. But be careful—"low fat" doesn't always mean low in calories. Sometimes extra sugars are added to low-fat desserts, for example.) For some women at very high risk, medication also may be necessary.

To develop a weight-loss or weight-maintenance program that works best for you, consult with your doctor, a registered dietitian, or a qualified nutritionist. For ideas on how to lose weight safely and keep it off, see "Aim for a Healthy Weight" on page 83.

Physical Inactivity

Physical inactivity raises your risk of heart disease—more than you might think. It boosts your chances of developing heart-related problems even if you have no other risk factors. It also increases the likelihood that you will develop other heart disease risk factors, such as high blood pressure, diabetes, and overweight. Lack of physical activity leads to more doctor visits, more hospitalizations, and use of medicines for a variety of illnesses.

Yet most women aren't getting enough physical activity. According to the Centers for Disease Control and Prevention, 60 percent of Americans are not meeting the recommended levels of physical activity. Fully 16 percent of Americans are not active at all. Overall, older people are less likely to be active than younger individuals, and women tend to be less physically active than men. Physical inactivity is especially common among African American and Hispanic women.

For women, physical inactivity also increases the risk of osteoporosis, which in turn may increase the risk of broken bones. This is worrisome, because women tend to become less physically active as they get older.

Fortunately, research shows that as little as 30 minutes of moderate activity on most, and preferably all, days of the week helps to protect your health. This level of activity can reduce your risk of heart disease as well as lower your chances of having a stroke, colon cancer, high blood pressure, diabetes, and other medical problems.

Examples of moderate activity are taking a brisk walk, raking leaves, dancing, light weightlifting, house cleaning, or gardening. If you prefer, you can divide your 30-minute activity into shorter periods of at least 10 minutes each. To find out about easy, enjoyable ways to boost your activity level, see "Learn New Moves" on page 94.

Diabetes

Diabetes is a major risk factor for heart disease and stroke. More than 65 percent of people who have diabetes die of some type of cardiovascular disease. Diabetic women are at especially high risk for dying of heart disease and stroke. Today, 7 million women in the United States have diabetes, including an estimated 3 million women who do not even know they have the disease.

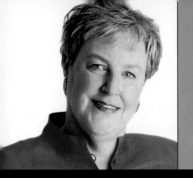

ANN

"I wasn't aware of my risk factors, such as being diabetic and having a family history of heart problems."

The type of diabetes that most commonly develops in adulthood is type 2 diabetes. In type 2 diabetes, the pancreas makes insulin, but the body cannot use it properly and gradually loses the ability to produce it. Type 2 diabetes is a serious disease. In addition to increasing the risk for heart disease, it is the #1 cause of kidney failure, blindness, and lower limb amputation in adults. Diabetes can also lead to nerve damage and difficulties in fighting infection.

The risk of type 2 diabetes rises after the age of 45. You are much more likely to develop this disease if you are overweight, especially if you have extra weight around your waist. Other risk factors include physical inactivity and a family history of diabetes. Type 2 diabetes also is more common among American Indians, Hispanic Americans, African Americans, Asian Americans, and Pacific Islanders. Women who have had diabetes during pregnancy (gestational diabetes) or have given birth to a baby weighing more than 9 pounds are also more likely to develop type 2 diabetes later in life.

Symptoms of diabetes may include fatigue, nausea, frequent urination, unusual thirst, weight loss, blurred vision, frequent infections, and slow healing of sores. But type 2 diabetes develops gradually and sometimes has no symptoms. Even if you have no symptoms of diabetes, if you are overweight and have any of the risk factors for type 2 diabetes, ask your doctor about getting tested for it. You have diabetes if your fasting blood glucose level is 126 mg/dL or higher.

If you have diabetes, controlling your blood glucose (blood sugar) levels will help to prevent complications. Because diabetes is so strongly linked with heart disease, managing diabetes must include keeping certain factors under control (See "The ABCs of Diabetes Control" on page 47.). Recommended levels of blood pressure and blood cholesterol control are lower for people with diabetes than for most others. Not smoking, being physically active, and taking aspirin daily (if your doctor recommends it) also are important ways to prevent heart disease if you have diabetes.

Some people do not yet have diabetes but are at high risk for developing the disease. They have a condition known as "prediabetes," in which blood glucose levels are higher than normal but not yet in the diabetic range. But new research shows that many people with prediabetes can prevent or delay the development of diabetes by making modest changes in diet and level of physical activity (See "Preventing Diabetes" on page 48.).

People who are prediabetic also have a 50 percent greater chance of having a heart attack or stroke than those who have normal blood glucose levels. If you are prediabetic, you'll need to pay close attention to preventing or controlling blood pressure, high blood cholesterol, and other risk factors for heart disease.

"AT THE TIME, IT NEVER OCCURRED
TO ME THAT I COULD BE HAVING
A HEART ATTACK. I THINK ABOUT
HEART DISEASE EVERY
DAY NOW."

—Sharon

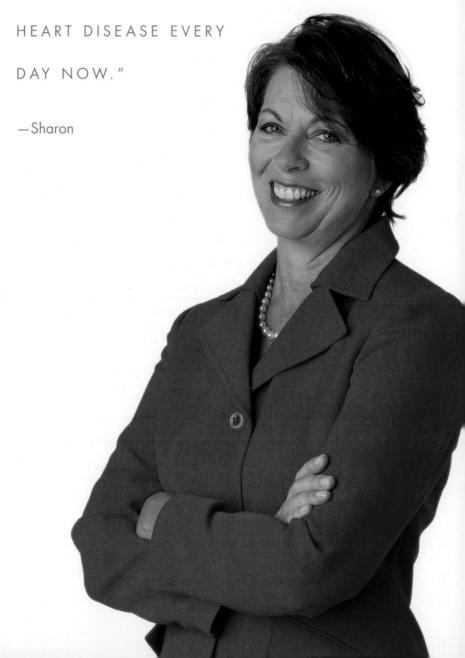

THE ABCs OF DIABETES *control*

If you have diabetes, three key steps can help you lower your risk of heart attack and stroke. Follow these **ABCs**:

A is for the **A1C test**, which is short for hemoglobin A1C. This test measures your average blood glucose (blood sugar) over the last 3 months. It lets you know if your blood glucose level is under control. Get this test at least twice a year. The number to aim for is below 7.

B is for **blood pressure**. The higher your blood pressure, the harder your heart has to work. Get your blood pressure measured at every doctor's visit. The numbers to aim for are below 130/80 mmHg.

C is for **cholesterol**. LDL, or "bad" cholesterol, builds up and clogs your arteries. Get your LDL cholesterol tested at least once a year. The number to aim for is below 100 mg/dL. Your doctor may advise you to aim for an even lower target number, for example, less than 70.

Be sure to ask your doctor these questions:
- What are my ABC numbers?
- What should my ABC target numbers be?
- What actions should I take to reach my ABC target numbers?

To lower your risk of heart attack and stroke, also take these steps:
- Be physically active every day.
- Follow your doctor's advice about the type of physical activity that's best for you.
- Eat less salt and sodium, saturated fat, *trans* fat, and cholesterol.
- Eat more fiber. Choose fiber-rich whole grains, fruits, vegetables, and beans.
- Stay at a healthy weight.
- If you smoke, stop.
- Take medicines as prescribed.
- Ask your doctor about taking aspirin.
- Ask others to help you manage your diabetes.

preventing DIABETES

If you have "prediabetes"—higher than normal glucose levels—you are more likely to develop type 2 diabetes. But you can take steps to improve your health and delay or possibly prevent diabetes. A recent study showed that many overweight, prediabetic people dramatically reduced the risk of developing diabetes by following a lower fat, lower calorie diet and getting 30 minutes of physical activity at least 5 days per week. The following are some encouraging results of the study:

- Overall, people who achieved a 5 to 7 percent weight loss (about 10 to 15 pounds) through diet and increased physical activity (usually brisk walking) reduced their risk of diabetes by 58 percent over the next 3 years.

- For people over age 60, these lifestyle changes reduced the risk of developing diabetes by 71 percent.

- Benefits were seen in all of the racial and ethnic groups who participated in the study—Caucasians, African Americans, Hispanics, American Indians, Asian Americans, and Pacific Islanders.

- People taking the diabetes drug metformin (Glucophage®) reduced their risk of developing the disease by 31 percent.

These findings suggest that you can act to prevent or delay diabetes, even if you are at high risk for the disease. For more information on how to choose and cook low-fat foods, get more physical activity, and achieve a healthy weight, see "Taking Control" on page 60.

OTHER FACTORS THAT *affect* HEART DISEASE

Menopausal Hormone Therapy: What Every Woman Needs To Know

Menopausal hormone therapy once seemed the answer for many of the conditions women face as they age. It was thought that hormone therapy could ward off heart disease, osteoporosis, and cancer, while improving women's quality of life.

But beginning in July 2002, findings emerged from clinical trials that showed this was not so. In fact, long-term use of hormone therapy poses serious risks and may increase the risk of heart attack and stroke.

The findings come from the Women's Health Initiative (WHI), launched in 1991 to test ways to prevent a number of medical disorders in postmenopausal women. It consists of a set of clinical studies on hormone therapy, diet modification, and calcium and vitamin D supplements; an observational study; and a community prevention study.

The two hormone therapy clinical studies were both stopped early because of serious risks and the failure to prevent heart disease. One of the hormone studies involved 16,608 postmenopausal women with a uterus who took either estrogen-plus-progestin therapy or a placebo. (The added progestin protects women against uterine cancer. A placebo is a substance that looks like the real drug but has no biologic effect.) The other study involved 10,739 women who had had a hysterectomy and took estrogen alone or a placebo. The estrogen used in the WHI was conjugated equine estrogens (0.625 mg daily), and the progestin was medroxyprogesterone acetate (2.5 mg daily).

In brief, the studies concluded the following:

Estrogen-plus-progestin therapy increased women's risk for heart attacks, stroke, blood clots, and breast cancer. It also doubled the risk of dementia and did not protect women against memory loss.

However, the estrogen-plus-progestin therapy had some benefits: It reduced the risk for colorectal cancer and fractures. It also relieved menopausal symptoms, such as hot flashes and night sweats, in women who suffered from them. But the study found that estrogen plus progestin did not improve women's overall quality of life.

Estrogen-alone therapy increased the risk for stroke and venous thrombosis (blood clot, usually in one of the deep veins of the legs). It had no effect on heart disease and colorectal cancer, and it did not increase the risk of breast cancer. Estrogen alone gave no protection against memory loss, and there were more cases of dementia in those who took the therapy than those on the placebo, although the increase was not statistically significant. Estrogen alone reduced the risk for fractures.

The research showed that both types of medication—estrogen alone and estrogen with progestin—increased the risk of developing urinary incontinence, which is the inability to "hold in" urine. For women who already have the condition, these medications can worsen symptoms.

If you are currently on or have taken menopausal hormone therapy, the findings can't help but concern you. It is important to know, however, that those results apply to a large group of women. An individual woman's increased risk for disease is quite small. For example, each woman in the estrogen-plus-progestin study had, on average, an increased risk of breast cancer of less than one-tenth of 1 percent per year.

While questions remain, these findings provide a basis for some advice about using hormone therapy:

- **Estrogen alone, or estrogen plus progestin**, should not be used to prevent heart disease. Talk with your doctor about other ways of preventing heart attack and stroke, including lifestyle changes and medicines such as cholesterol-lowering statins and blood pressure drugs.

- If you are considering using menopausal hormone therapy to prevent osteoporosis, talk with your doctor about the possible benefits weighed against your personal risks for heart attack, stroke, blood clots, and breast cancer. Ask your doctor about alternative treatments that are safe and effective in preventing osteoporosis and bone fractures.

- Do not take menopausal hormone therapy to prevent dementia or memory loss.

- If you are considering menopausal hormone therapy to provide relief from menopausal symptoms such as hot flashes, talk with your doctor about whether this treatment is right for you. The WHI did not test the short-term risks and benefits of using hormone therapy for menopausal symptoms. The U.S. Food and Drug Administration recommends that menopausal hormone therapy be used at the lowest dose for the shortest period of time to reach treatment goals.

And remember, your risk for heart disease, stroke, osteoporosis, and other conditions may change as you age, so review your health regularly with your doctor. New treatments that are safe and effective may become available. Stay informed. If you have heart disease, see page 53 for more on menopausal hormone therapy.

Stress and Depression

Many women are concerned about a possible connection between stress and heart disease. Many studies do report a connection for both women and men. For example, the most commonly reported "trigger" for a heart attack is an emotionally upsetting event, particularly one involving anger. After a heart attack, people with higher levels of stress and anxiety tend to have more trouble recovering. Also, some common ways of coping with stress, such as overeating, heavy drinking, and smoking, are clearly bad for your heart.

But stress is not the only emotional influence on heart health. Depression, too, is common in both women and men after a heart attack or heart surgery. If you have had a heart attack or heart surgery and find yourself feeling depressed or "blue" for a long time afterward, or if the sad feelings are severe, talk with your doctor about ways to get help. Also keep in mind that support from family, friends, and other heart patients can help to improve mood and adjustment to the recovery process.

The good news is that sensible health habits can have a protective effect. Regular physical activity not only relieves stress and depression but also can directly lower your risk of heart disease. Research also shows that participating in a stress management program after a heart attack lessens the chances of further heart-related problems. Stress management programs, as well as support groups for heart patients, can also help you develop new ways of handling everyday life challenges.

Good relationships count, too. Developing strong personal ties reduces the chances of developing heart disease. Supportive relationships also help to prolong people's lives after a heart attack. Religious or spiritual beliefs and activity are also linked to longer survival among heart surgery patients.

CAN YOUNGER *women* SAFELY TAKE ESTROGEN THERAPY?

You may have read media reports of updated WHI findings suggesting that estrogen-alone therapy may protect younger postmenopausal women from heart disease. Does this mean that women in their 50s should start taking estrogen to protect their hearts? The answer is still no. Here are the facts:

Researchers examined health outcomes for women in the WHI study who had undergone hysterectomies and had taken estrogen-alone therapy. For older women (ages 60 to 79) in the study, taking estrogen offered no overall protection from heart attack or coronary death. But among a subgroup of women ages 50 to 59, there was a suggestion of lower coronary heart disease risk. What do these findings mean for you?

- If you are considering using short-term estrogen-alone therapy around the time of menopause, for the relief of hot flashes and other temporary symptoms, these findings may be somewhat reassuring.

- But keep in mind that estrogen-alone therapy—the medication used in this study—is appropriate only for women who have had hysterectomies. Other women cannot use it, because it can cause uterine cancer.

- This study does not change the overall conclusion from the WHI: Hormones should not be used for the prevention of coronary heart disease at any age. Hormone therapy has many other risks, including stroke and blood clots. There are far safer and more effective ways to protect your heart.

"SINCE THE HEART ATTACK, I TRY TO WALK AT LEAST 4 MILES A DAY AND AVOID FOODS HIGH IN CHOLESTEROL, SALT, SUGAR, AND FAT. I KNOW HOW IMPORTANT HEART HEALTH IS, SO I TRY TO PASS THIS KNOWLEDGE AND HEALTHY LIFESTYLE ON TO MY KIDS." —Maria

"WATCHING MY MOM DEAL WITH HEART DISEASE HAS TAUGHT ME TO BE MINDFUL OF WHAT I DO EVERY DAY." —Christen

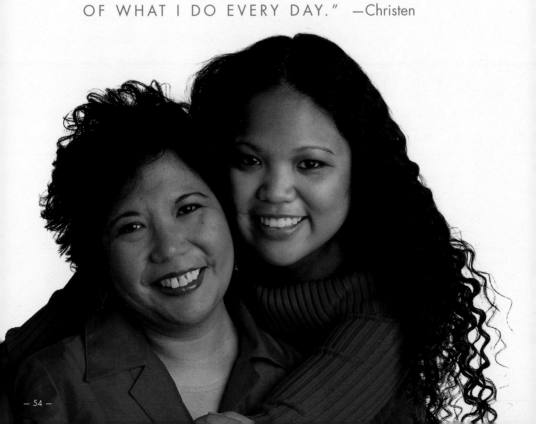

Much remains to be learned about the connections among stress, depression, and heart disease, but a few things are clear: staying physically active, developing a wide circle of supportive people in your life, and sharing your feelings and concerns with them can help you to be happier and live longer.

Alcohol

Recent research suggests that moderate drinkers are less likely to develop heart disease than people who don't drink any alcohol or who drink too much. Small amounts of alcohol may help protect against heart disease by raising levels of HDL "good" cholesterol.

If you are a nondrinker, this is not a recommendation to start using alcohol. Recent studies show that alcohol use increases the risk of breast cancer. And, certainly, if you are pregnant, planning to become pregnant, or have another health condition that could make alcohol use harmful, you should not drink. Otherwise, if you're already a moderate drinker, you may be less likely to have a heart attack.

It is important, though, to weigh benefits against risks. Talk with your doctor about your personal risks of breast cancer, heart disease, and other health conditions that may be affected by drinking alcohol. With the help of your doctor, decide whether moderate drinking to lower heart attack risk outweighs the possible increased risk of breast cancer or other medical problems.

If you do decide to use alcohol, remember that moderation is the key. Heavy drinking causes many heart-related problems. More than three drinks per day can raise blood pressure and triglyceride levels, while binge drinking can contribute to stroke. Too much alcohol also can damage the heart muscle, leading to heart failure. Overall, people who drink heavily on a regular basis have higher rates of heart disease than either moderate drinkers or nondrinkers.

WHAT IS *moderate* DRINKING?

For women, moderate drinking is defined as no more than one drink per day, according to the "Dietary Guidelines for Americans." Count the following as one drink:

- 12 ounces of beer (150 calories)
- 5 ounces of wine (100 calories)
- 1¹/₂ ounces of 80-proof distilled spirits (100 calories)

Birth Control Pills

Studies show that women who use high-dose birth control pills (oral contraceptives) are more likely to have a heart attack or stroke because blood clots are more likely to form in the blood vessels. These risks are lessened once the birth control pill is stopped. Using the pill also may worsen the effects of other risk factors, such as smoking, high blood pressure, diabetes, high blood cholesterol, and overweight.

Much of this information comes from studies of birth control pills containing higher doses of hormones than those commonly used today. Still, the risks of using low-dose pills are not fully known. Therefore, if you are now taking any kind of birth control pill or are considering using one, keep these guidelines in mind:

Don't mix smoking and "the pill." If you smoke cigarettes, make a serious effort to quit. If you cannot quit, choose a different form of birth control. Cigarette smoking boosts the risk of serious health problems from birth control pill use, especially the risk of blood clots. For women over the age of 35, the risk is particularly high. Women who use birth control pills should not smoke.

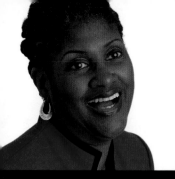

Pay attention to diabetes. Levels of glucose, or blood sugar, sometimes change dramatically in women who take birth control pills. Any woman who is diabetic or has a close relative who is diabetic should have regular blood sugar tests if she takes birth control pills.

Watch your blood pressure. After starting to take birth control pills, your blood pressure may go up. If your blood pressure increases to 140/90 mmHg or higher, ask your doctor about changing pills or switching to another form of birth control. Be sure to get your blood pressure checked at least once a year.

Talk with your doctor. If you have heart disease or another heart problem, or if you have suffered a stroke, birth control pills may not be a safe choice. Be sure your doctor knows about these or other serious health conditions before prescribing birth control pills for you.

Sleep Apnea

Sleep apnea is a serious disorder in which a person briefly and repeatedly stops breathing during sleep. People with untreated sleep apnea are more likely to develop high blood pressure, heart attack, congestive heart failure, and stroke.

Women are more likely to develop sleep apnea after menopause. Other factors that increase risk are overweight and obesity, smoking, the use of alcohol or sleeping pills, and a family history of sleep apnea. Symptoms include heavy snoring and gasping or choking during sleep, along with extreme daytime sleepiness.

If you think you may have sleep apnea, ask your doctor for a test called polysomnography, which is usually performed overnight in a sleep center. If you are overweight, even a small weight loss—10 percent of your current weight—can relieve mild cases of sleep apnea. Other self-help treatments include quitting smoking and avoiding alcohol and sleeping pills. Sleeping on your side rather than on your back also may help. Some people benefit from a mechanical device that helps maintain a regular breathing pattern by increasing air pressure through the nasal passages via a face mask. For very serious cases, surgery may be needed.

NEW RISK *factors?*

We know that major risk factors such as high blood cholesterol, high blood pressure, and smoking boost heart disease risk. Researchers are studying other factors that might contribute to heart disease, including inflammation of the artery walls. Several emerging risk factors have been identified. We don't know for sure yet whether they lead to heart disease or whether treating them will reduce risk. Although these possible risk factors are not recommended for routine testing, ask your doctor whether you should be tested for any of them.

C-reactive protein (CRP). High levels of CRP may indicate inflammation in the artery walls. A simple blood test can measure the levels of CRP in the blood. In many cases, a high CRP level is a sign of metabolic syndrome. Treatment of the syndrome with lifestyle changes—weight loss and regular physical activity—can often lower CRP.

Homocysteine. High blood levels of this amino acid may increase risk for heart disease. For women, homocysteine levels tend to rise after menopause. It may be possible to lower elevated levels of homocysteine by getting plenty of folic acid and vitamins B6 and B12 in your diet.

Lp(a) protein. This lipoprotein may make it easier for blood clots to form. Niacin, a cholesterol-lowering drug, may help to lower Lp(a) protein levels.

TAKING *control*

*N*ow that you know the risks for heart disease, what can you do to protect yourself? The good news: plenty. Research shows that women can lower their heart disease risk enormously—by as much as 82 percent—simply by leading a healthy lifestyle. This section will offer dozens of down-to-earth ideas for making heart healthy practices part of your daily life.

If you already have heart disease, this section also will tell you about the kinds of tests, treatments, and medications that can help you stay healthier. You will also find out about the warning signs of a heart attack and how to get fast, life-saving help.

For all women, choosing a healthy lifestyle is extremely important. Remember, heart disease is a woman's greatest health threat. Adopting heart healthy habits can add years to your life—vital, active years. Research from the Framingham Heart Study shows that women who have no risk factors for heart disease live an average of 8 years longer than women with two or more risk factors.

Sometimes, women are so good at taking care of others that they don't take the time to keep themselves healthy and strong. Make time to take care of yourself. Making healthy changes in your daily habits will give you more energy and stamina to enjoy the people and activities you love. And once you get started, keep it up. Ask your family and friends to support you in maintaining your new, heart healthy lifestyle. You're worth it!

Research shows that women can lower their heart disease risk enormously—by as much as 82 percent—simply by leading a healthy lifestyle.

A FAMILY PLAN FOR HEART *health*

*W*hen it comes to heart health, what's good for you is good for your whole family—including its youngest members. We now know that two-thirds of teenagers have at least one risk factor for heart disease, from overweight and "couch potato-itis" to unhealthy blood pressure and cholesterol levels. Even more disturbing, about 1 million U.S. teens have metabolic syndrome, a cluster of risk factors that greatly increases the risk of a later heart attack. By teaching your children, grandchildren, or other young family members the importance of eating well and getting regular physical activity, you'll help them develop healthy habits for a lifetime. Here are some ways to get started:

Set a good example. Adults have a big influence on children's and teens' behavior—even though kids may not want to admit it! If you follow a healthy lifestyle, younger family members will be more likely to do the same. Let them see you eating nutritious snacks and enjoying outdoor activities. Invite them to join you.

Raise "kitchen kids." Show young children how to clean fruits and veggies and combine them into salads. When they are old enough, teach them to use the cooktop, oven, microwave, and toaster safely. Show teens how to make simple, healthy dishes, such as pasta with vegetables and broiled chicken or fish. Children who have basic cooking skills appreciate food more and are more likely to try new dishes.

Get them moving. Encourage your kids or grandkids to get some exercise throughout the day and especially on weekends. Go on outings with them that involve activities such as hiking, swimming, or bicycling. Walk, bike, or jog with them to places close by. Use your backyard or local park for basketball, baseball, football, badminton, or volleyball.

AN ACTION PLAN FOR *heart* HEALTH

*H*ere's *The Heart Truth*: If you eat a nutritious diet, engage in regular physical activity, maintain a healthy weight, and stop smoking, you will improve your heart health. Currently, only 3 percent of U.S. adults practice these "Big Four" heart healthy habits. But it's never too late to start. No matter what heart disease risk factors you have—or how many—you will greatly benefit from taking action in these four areas. If you already have heart disease, you can lessen its severity by following this plan.

True, you may need to take other steps to prevent or control heart disease. For example, if you have diabetes, you also will need to keep your blood sugar levels under control. But following a heart healthy eating plan, controlling your weight, and engaging in more physical activity will help you keep your blood sugar at healthy levels. These steps will also help reduce your chances of developing high blood pressure or high blood cholesterol. Whatever your current health conditions or habits, this action plan can make an enormously positive difference in your heart health. To find out how to get started, read on.

Eat for Health

The health of your heart has a lot to do with the foods you eat. The "Dietary Guidelines for Americans" give science-based advice for eating right and being physically active to maintain good health. The guidelines recommend the following healthy eating plans:

- Emphasize fruits, vegetables, whole grains, and fat-free or low-fat milk and milk products.

- Include lean meats, poultry, fish, beans, eggs, and nuts.

- Choose foods that are low in saturated fats, *trans* fats, cholesterol, salt and sodium, and added sugars.

- Balance the calories you take in with the calories you need.

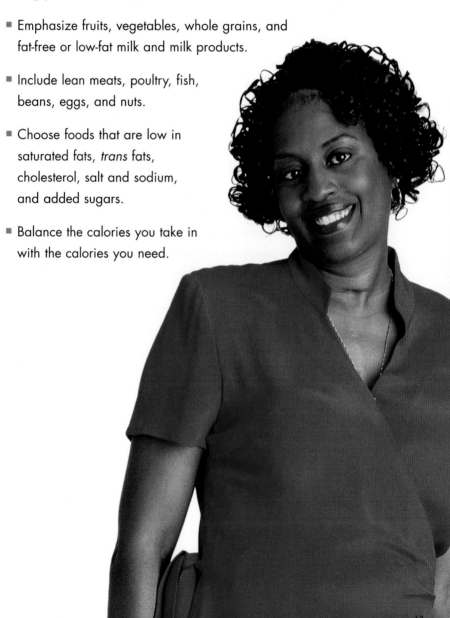

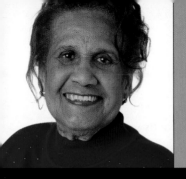

OLGA

"To keep my condition under control I make sure to follow my doctor's advice, take prescriptions, and get treatment when I need it."

Although the "Dietary Guidelines for Americans" recommend an excellent basic menu for heart health, you may need to make some additional changes in your diet if you have high blood pressure or high blood cholesterol. You may want to work with a registered dietitian to help you make these changes. A dietitian can teach you about the eating plan that is best for you, determine a reasonable calorie level, and help you choose foods and plan menus. A dietitian can also help you keep track of your progress and encourage you to stay on your eating plan. Talk with your doctor about whether you should get a referral to a registered dietitian. In the meantime, if you have high blood pressure or high blood cholesterol, the following page has some guidelines.

HOW TO READ A NUTRITIONAL FACTS LABEL

Macaroni & Cheese

Start Here →

Check Calories

Limit These Nutrients

Get Enough of These Nutrients

Footnote

Nutrition Facts

Serving Size 1 cup (228g)
Servings Per Container 2

Amount Per Serving

Calories 250   Calories from Fat 110

                                    % Daily Value*

Total Fat 12g	**18%**
Saturated Fat 3g	**15%**
Trans Fat 3g	
Cholesterol 30mg	**10%**
Sodium 470mg	**20%**
Total Carbohydrate 31g	**10%**
Dietary Fiber 0g	**0%**
Sugars 5g	
Protein 5g	

Vitamin A	4%
Vitamin C	2%
Calcium	20%
Iron	4%

* Percent Daily Values are based on a 2,000 calorie diet. Your Daily values may be higher or lower depending on your calorie needs.

	Calories:	2,000	2,500
Total Fat	Less Than	65g	80g
Sat Fat	Less Than	20g	25g
Cholosteral	Less Than	300mg	300mg
Sodium	Less than	2,400mg	2,400mg
Total Carbohydrate		300g	375g
Dietary Fiber		25g	30g

Quick Guide to % Daily Value

- **5% or Less Is Low**

- **20% or More Is High**

Blood Pressure and the DASH Eating Plan

If you have high blood pressure or prehypertension, you may want to follow an eating plan called "DASH." DASH stands for "Dietary Approaches to Stop Hypertension," and the DASH eating plan emphasizes fruits, vegetables, fat-free or low-fat milk and milk products, whole grain products, fish, poultry, beans, seeds, and nuts. The DASH eating plan also contains less salt/sodium, sweets, added sugars, sugar containing beverages, fats, and red meats than the typical American diet. This heart healthy way of eating is also lower in saturated fat and cholesterol and is rich in nutrients that are associated with lowering blood pressure—mainly potassium, magnesium, calcium, protein, and fiber.

A major study found that people who followed this eating plan reduced their blood pressure more than those who ate more "typical" American diets, which have fewer fruits and vegetables. A second study found that people who followed the DASH eating plan and cut down on sodium had the biggest reductions in blood pressure. (Salt, or sodium chloride, and other forms of sodium are found in many processed foods.) So, for a truly winning combination, follow the DASH eating plan and lower your sodium intake as much as possible. The study found that the less sodium people consumed, the more their blood pressure dropped.

The DASH eating plan is geared especially to people with high blood pressure or prehypertension, but it is a healthy plan for anyone, so share it with your family. When people who have normal blood pressure follow the DASH eating plan, especially when they also consume less sodium, they may lessen their chances of developing high blood pressure. Remember, 90 percent of middle-aged Americans go on to develop high blood pressure. Use the DASH plan to help beat the odds!

"I HAVE TO LOSE WEIGHT AND REDUCE MY

CHOLESTEROL. THIS IS JUST THE BEGINNING

OF A LONG BATTLE, AND

I KNOW IT WON'T

BE EASY, BUT I KNOW

I HAVE TO DO IT."

—Rosario

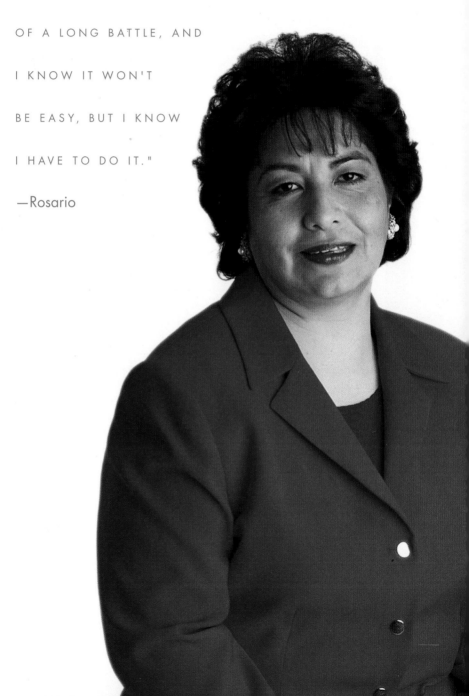

THE DASH EATING PLAN

The DASH eating plan shown below is based on 2,000 calories a day. The number of daily servings in a food group may vary from those listed, depending on how many daily calories you need.

Food Group	Daily Servings (except as noted)	Serving Sizes
Grains*	6–8	1 slice bread 1 oz dry cereal† 1/2 cup cooked rice, pasta, or cereal
Vegetables	4–5	1 cup raw leafy vegetables 1/2 cup cooked vegetables 6 oz vegetable juice
Fruits	4–5	1 medium fruit 1/4 cup dried fruit 1/2 cup fresh, frozen, or canned fruit 1/2 cup fruit juice
Low-fat or fat-free milk and milk products	2–3	1 cup milk or yogurt 1 1/2 oz cheese
Lean meats, poultry, and fish	6 or less	1 oz cooked meats, poultry, or fish 1 egg‡
Nuts, seeds, and legumes	4–5 per week	1/3 cup or 1 1/2 oz nuts 2 tbsp peanut butter 2 tbsp or 1/2 oz seeds 1/2 cup cooked legumes (dry beans and peas)

Food Group	Daily Servings (except as noted)	Serving Sizes
Fats and oils§	2–3	1 tsp soft margarine 1 tsp vegetable oil 1 tbsp mayonnaise 2 tbsp light salad dressing
Sweets and added sugars	5 or less per week	1 tbsp sugar 1 tbsp jelly or jam $1/2$ cup sorbet or gelatin 1 cup lemonade

* Whole grains are recommended for most grain servings as a good source of fiber and nutrients.

† Serving sizes vary between $1/2$ cup and $1 1/4$ cups. Check the product's Nutrition Facts label.

‡ Since eggs are high in cholesterol, limit egg yolks to no more than four per week. Two egg whites have the same amount of protein as 1 ounce of meat.

§ Fat content changes the serving amount for fats and oils. For example, 1 tbsp of regular salad dressing equals 1 serving; 1 tbsp of a low-fat dressing equals one-half serving; 1 tbsp of a fat-free dressing equals zero servings.

HOLD THE SALT: HOW TO *reduce* SALT AND SODIUM IN YOUR DIET

You can help prevent and control high blood pressure by cutting down on salt and other forms of sodium. Try to consume no more than 2,300 mg of sodium a day—or, if you can, no more than 1,500 mg a day (2,300 mg of sodium equals 1 tsp of table salt, while 1,500 mg equals $^2/_3$ tsp). Here are some tips on limiting your intake of salt and sodium:

- Choose low-sodium, reduced-sodium, or no-salt-added versions of foods and condiments, when available.

- Choose fresh, frozen, or canned (low-sodium or no-salt-added) vegetables.

- Use fresh poultry, fish, and lean meat, rather than canned, smoked, or processed types.

- Choose ready-to-eat breakfast cereals that are lower in sodium.

- Limit cured foods (such as bacon and ham), foods packed in brine (such as pickles, pickled vegetables, olives, and sauerkraut), and condiments (such as mustard, horseradish, ketchup, and barbeque sauce). Limit even lower sodium versions of soy sauce and teriyaki sauce. Use these condiments sparingly, as you do table salt.

- Cook rice, pasta, and hot cereals without salt. Cut back on instant or flavored rice, pasta, and cereal mixes, which usually have added salt.

- Choose "convenience foods" that are lower in sodium. Cut back on frozen dinners, mixed dishes such as pizza, packaged mixes, canned soups or broths, and salad dressings. These foods often have a lot of sodium.

- Rinse canned foods, such as tuna and canned beans, to remove some of the sodium.

- Salt substitutes containing potassium chloride may be useful for some individuals, but they can be harmful to people with certain medical conditions. Ask your doctor before trying salt substitutes.

- When you cook, be "spicy" instead of "salty." In cooking and at the table, flavor foods with herbs, spices, wine, lemon, lime, vinegar, or salt-free seasoning blends. Start by cutting your salt use in half.

What Else Affects Blood Pressure?

A number of foods and other factors have been reported to affect blood pressure. Here are the latest research findings:

- **Garlic and onions.** These foods have not been found to affect blood pressure, but they are tasty, nutritious substitutes for salty seasonings and can be used often.

- **Caffeine.** This may cause blood pressure to rise, but only temporarily. Unless you are sensitive to caffeine, you do not have to limit how much you consume to prevent or control high blood pressure.

- **Stress.** Stress, too, can make blood pressure go up for a while and has been thought to contribute to high blood pressure. But the long-term effects of stress are not clear. Furthermore, stress management techniques do not seem to prevent high blood pressure. However, stress management may help you to control other unhealthy habits, such as smoking, overeating, or using too much alcohol.

High Blood Cholesterol and the TLC Program

The TLC Program can help you to lower high blood cholesterol and protect your health. TLC stands for "Therapeutic Lifestyle Changes," a program that includes an eating plan that is low in saturated fat, *trans* fat, and cholesterol. The eating plan also adds plant stanols and sterols to your diet as well as more soluble fiber. The TLC Program also calls for increased physical activity and weight control. Adopt the TLC Program and you'll lower your chances of developing heart disease, future heart attacks, and other heart disease complications. (The main difference between the TLC and the DASH eating plans is that the TLC plan puts more emphasis on decreasing saturated fat and *trans* fat to lower blood cholesterol levels.)

eating THE TLC WAY

If your LDL cholesterol is above your goal level (see pages 32 and 33), you should start on the TLC eating plan right away. The TLC eating plan will help to reduce your LDL cholesterol and lower your chances of developing heart disease. If you already have heart disease, it will lessen your chances of a heart attack and other heart-related problems. On the TLC eating plan, you should eat as follows:

- Less than 7 percent of the day's total calories from saturated fat. Lowering saturated fat is the most important dietary change for reducing blood cholesterol.

- Less than 200 mg of dietary cholesterol a day.

- No more than 25 to 35 percent of daily calories from total fat (includes saturated fat calories).

- Just enough calories to reach or maintain a healthy weight.

- In addition, you should get at least 30 minutes of moderate-intensity physical activity on most, and preferably all, days of the week.

If your blood cholesterol is not lowered enough on the TLC Program, your doctor or registered dietitian may advise you to increase the amount of soluble fiber and/or add cholesterol-lowering food products. These products include margarines that contain ingredients called "plant sterols" or "plant stanol esters," which lower LDL cholesterol. If your LDL level is still not lowered enough, your doctor may prescribe a cholesterol-lowering drug along with the TLC Program. (See "To Learn More" on page 121.)

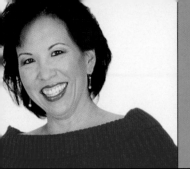

PATTIE

"There are a lot of things I want to do in my life, so I know it's important to take care of my health. Most women put everyone else before themselves, but you can't put off taking care of your heart."

The Lowdown on Low Fat

Recently, a large study reported what seemed to be startling results: women who reduced their total fat intake did not significantly reduce their risks for heart disease and other serious disorders. This widely publicized Women's Health Initiative (WHI) study, which tracked more than 48,000 postmenopausal women, found that those who ate lower fat diets for an average of 8 years had about the same risk of heart attack, stroke, breast cancer, and colon cancer as did women who ate whatever they wanted.

Does this mean we can feast on french fries and fudge without a second thought? Not at all. The WHI study was designed to study the impact of reducing total fat, without distinguishing between "good" fats found in fish, nuts, and vegetable oils, and "bad" fats like saturated fat and *trans* fat, which are found in processed foods, meats, and some dairy products. The type of fat you eat affects your heart disease risk. Other studies have found that reducing "bad" fats lowers risks for heart disease and future heart attacks, while consuming small amounts of "good" fats may be protective. In fact, a closer look at the WHI study supports the heart benefits of reducing "bad" fats.

The bottom line is that women should continue to follow an eating plan that is low in saturated fat, *trans* fat, and cholesterol to reduce their risk of heart disease. (For specifics, see "Figuring Out Fat" on page 81.) Most of the fat you consume each day should come from vegetable oils, fish, nuts, and other sources of polyunsaturated and monosaturated fats.

Now You're Cooking: Limiting Saturated Fat,
Trans Fat, and Cholesterol

Planning and preparing nutritious meals may take a little extra
effort, but the health benefits are huge. Here are some tips for
cutting down on saturated fat, *trans* fat, and dietary cholesterol,
which will help to lower your LDL cholesterol and reduce your
heart disease risk. It will improve heart health for all women, and
may be particularly helpful for those following the TLC eating plan.

Meat, Poultry, and Fish

- Choose fish, poultry, and lean cuts of meat. Trim the fat from
  meats; remove the skin and fat from chicken. Keep portion
  sizes moderate.

- Broil, bake, roast, or poach instead of frying. When you do fry,
  use a nonstick pan and a nonstick cooking spray or a very small
  amount of oil or margarine.

- Cut down on sausage, bacon, and processed high-fat cold cuts
  (which are also high in sodium).

Milk Products and Eggs

- Instead of whole milk or cream, use fat-free or 1-percent milk.

- Use fat-free or low-fat cheeses and yogurt.

- Replace ice cream with sorbet, sherbet, and fat-free or low-fat
  frozen yogurt. Keep portion sizes moderate.

- Limit the number of egg yolks you eat. Two or fewer yolks per
  week—including yolks in baked goods and in cooked or
  processed foods. Egg whites contain no fat or cholesterol, so
  you can eat them often. In most recipes, you can substitute
  two egg whites for one whole egg.

- Use soft margarines (liquid or tub types) that contain little or no
  trans fat. *Trans* fat is another type of dietary fat that raises LDL
  cholesterol.

Grains and Grain Products

- Eat foods with lots of fiber and nutrients and make sure that at least half of your grain products are whole grain. These include whole-grain breads, pastas, and cereals, as well as brown rice. When you check package labels, look for the word "whole" in the ingredients. Make sure that whole grains appear among the first items listed.

Sauces, Soups, and Casseroles

- After making sauces or soups, cool them in the refrigerator and skim the fat from the top. Do the same with canned soups.

- Thicken a low-fat sauce with cornstarch or flour.

- Make main dishes with whole-grain pasta, rice, or dry peas and beans. If you add meat, use small pieces for flavoring rather than as the main ingredient.

When You Can't Face Cooking

- Check nutrition labels to choose frozen dinners and pizzas that are lowest in saturated fat, *trans* fat, and cholesterol. Make sure the dinners include vegetables, fruits, and whole grains— or add them on the side.

- Choose store-bought baked goods that are lowest in saturated fat, cholesterol, *trans* fats, and hydrogenated (hardened) fats. *Trans* fats, or *trans* fatty acids, are formed when vegetable oil is hardened to become margarine or shortening in a process called "hydrogenation." Foods high in *trans* fats tend to raise blood cholesterol. Read labels. To reduce *trans* fats, limit products that list "hydrogenated oil" or "partially hydrogenated oil" as an ingredient. Also, remember that even no cholesterol and fat-free baked goods still may be high in calories.

Dining Out for Health

With a little planning—and a willingness to speak up—you can eat healthfully when you dine out. Here are some tips:

- You're the customer. Ask for what you want. Most restaurants will honor your requests. You have nothing to lose by asking!

- Order small. To reduce portion sizes, try ordering heart healthy appetizers or children's portions as your main meal. Or, take half of your entree home with you for lunch the next day.

- Ask questions. Don't hesitate to ask your server how foods are prepared and whether the restaurant will make substitutions. Ask if they will:

  - Serve low-fat or fat-free milk rather than whole milk or cream.

  - Tell you the type of cooking oil used. (Preferred types, which are lower in saturated fat, are canola, safflower, sunflower, corn, and olive oils.)

  - Trim visible fat off poultry or meat.

  - Leave all butter, gravy, and sauces off an entree or side dish.

  - Serve salad dressing on the side.

  - Meet special requests if you make them in advance.

- Select foods cooked by low-fat methods. Look for terms such as broiled, baked, roasted, poached, or lightly sauteed.

- Limit foods high in calories and fats, especially saturated fat and *trans* fat. Watch out for terms such as fried, crispy, creamed, escalloped, Hollandaise, Bearnaise, casserole, and pastry crust.

Make Healthy Choices For:

- **Breakfast:** Fresh fruit, a small glass of citrus juice, low-fat or fat-free milk and yogurt, whole-grain bread products and cereals, or an omelet made with egg whites or egg substitute.

- **Beverages:** Water with lemon, flavored sparkling water, juice spritzer (half fruit juice and half sparkling water), unsweetened iced tea, or reduced-sodium tomato juice.

- **Breads:** Most yeast breads are low in calories and fat—as long as you limit the butter, margarine, or olive oil. Choose whole-grain breads, which are packed with important nutrients and are full of fiber to make you feel fuller faster. Also, watch the sodium content.

- **Appetizers:** Steamed seafood, fresh fruit, bean soups, or salad with reduced-fat dressing.

- **Entrees:** Skinless poultry, fish, shellfish, vegetable dishes, or pasta with red sauce or vegetables. Limit your use of butter, margarine, and salt at the table.

- **Salads:** Fresh lettuce, spinach, and other greens; other fresh vegetables, chickpeas, and kidney beans. Skip high-fat and high-calorie nonvegetable choices such as deli meats, bacon, egg, cheese, and croutons. Choose lower calorie, reduced-fat, or fat-free dressings, lemon juice, or vinegar.

- **Side dishes:** Vegetables and grain products, including whole-grain rice or noodles. Ask for salsa or low-fat yogurt instead of sour cream or butter.

- **Dessert:** Fresh fruit, fat-free frozen yogurt, sherbet, or fruit sorbet (usually fat-free, but ask for the calorie content). Try sharing a dessert. If you drink coffee or tea with dessert, ask for low-fat or fat-free milk instead of cream or half-and-half.

LABEL LANGUAGE

Food labels can help you choose items that are lower in sodium, saturated and total fat, *trans* fat, cholesterol, and calories. When you shop for groceries, look for these claims on cans, bottles, and other packaging:

Sodium claims	What they mean
Sodium free or salt free	Less than 5 mg of sodium per serving
Very low sodium	35 mg or less per serving
Low sodium	140 mg or less per serving
Low-sodium meal	140 mg or less per 3 $1/2$ oz
Reduced or less sodium	At least 25% less than the regular version
Light in sodium	50% less than the regular version
Unsalted or no salt added	No salt added to product during processing, but this is not a sodium-free food
Fat claims	**What they mean**
Fat free	Less than $1/2$ g of fat per serving
Low saturated fat	1 g or less per serving and 15% or less of calories from saturated fat
Low fat	3 g or less per serving
Reduced fat	At least 25% less fat than the regular version
Light in fat	Half the fat compared to the regular version
Calorie claims	**What they mean**
Calorie free	Less than 5 calories per serving
Low calorie	40 calories or less per serving
Reduced or less calories	At least 25% fewer calories per serving than the regular version
Light or lite	50% less fat or 33% fewer calories than the regular version

Know Your Foods

The following are some additional tips on shopping, cooking, and eating for heart health:

- To choose foods wisely, see "How To Read a Nutritional Facts Label" on page 65 and "Label Language" on page 79.

- To prepare and eat heart healthy meals, see "Figuring Out Fat" on the next page and "What's in a Serving?" on page 82.

- For other tips on making good food choices, see "Healthy Snacking" below and "Vitamins for Heart Health" on page 84.

Healthy Snacking

Many snacks, including many types of cookies, crackers, and chips, are high in saturated fat, *trans* fat, cholesterol, sodium, and calories. But that doesn't mean you have to cut out all between-meal treats. Keep the foods listed below on hand for snack attacks. But keep in mind that while these snacks may be low in fat, many are not low in calories. So watch how much you eat, especially if you are trying to control your weight. Here are some healthier, low-fat snacks:

- 100-percent fruit juices

- Vegetable sticks; try a dab of reduced-fat peanut butter on celery sticks

- Fat-free frozen yogurt, sherbet, and sorbet

- Low-fat cookies, such as animal crackers, graham crackers, ginger snaps, and fig bars

- Low-fat crackers, such as melba toast, or rice, rye, and soda crackers. Look for unsalted or low-sodium types

- Air-popped popcorn with no salt or butter; fat-free, low-sodium pretzels

- Fresh or dried fruit or fruits canned in their own juice

FIGURING OUT FAT

Your personal "fat allowance" depends on how many calories you consume each day. If you do not have high blood cholesterol or heart disease, the saturated fat in your diet should be less than 10 percent of your daily calories, and total fat should be 20 to 35 percent of calories. Most fats should come from foods that are high in polyunsaturated fats and monosaturated fats, such as fish, nuts, and vegetable oils.

The table below shows the maximum amount of saturated fat you should eat, depending on how many calories you take in each day. If you have high blood cholesterol or heart disease, the amount of saturated fat will be different. (See "Eating the TLC Way" on page 73.) Check the Nutrition Facts panel on food labels to find out the number of fat grams—both saturated and total—in each serving.

Total Calorie Intake	Limit on Saturated Fat Intake
1,200	13 g or less
1,600	18 g or less
2,000*	20 g or less
2,200	24 g or less
2,500*	25 g or less
2,800	31 g or less

* Percent Daily Values on Nutrition Facts labels are based on a 2,000-calorie diet. Values for 2,000 and 2,500 calories are rounded to the nearest 5 gram to be consistent with the Nutrition Facts label.

WHAT'S IN A SERVING?

The "Dietary Guidelines for Americans" offer a healthy overall eating plan. But what counts as a serving? Here's a quick rundown of the food groups and number of servings you need of each:

Food Group/Daily Servings	What Counts as a Serving
Breads, cereals, rice, and pasta: 6–11 servings	1 slice bread 1 cup ready-to-eat cereal flakes $^1/_2$ cup cooked cereal, rice, pasta
Vegetables: 3–5 servings	1 cup raw leafy vegetables $^1/_2$ cup other vegetables $^3/_4$ cup of vegetable juice
Fruits: 2–4 servings	1 medium apple, banana, orange, pear $^1/_2$ cup fruit—chopped, cooked, canned $^3/_4$ cup fruit juice
Milk, yogurt, and cheese: 2–3 servings	1 cup milk (nonfat or low fat) 1 cup low-fat yogurt $1^1/_2$ oz low-fat natural cheese 2 oz low-fat processed cheese 1 cup soy-based beverage with added calcium
Meat, poultry, fish, dry beans, eggs, and nuts: 2–3 servings (totals 5–7 ounces per day)	2–3 oz of cooked lean meat, poultry, or fish $^1/_2$ cup of cooked dry beans or tofu counts as 1 oz of lean meat $2^1/_2$ oz soyburger or 1 egg counts as 1 oz of lean meat 2 tbsp of peanut butter or $^1/_3$ cup of nuts counts as 1 oz of meat
Fats, oils, and sweets	Use sparingly. Choose foods lower in fat, saturated fat, *trans* fat, and cholesterol

Aim for a Healthy Weight

If you are overweight or obese, taking off pounds can reduce your chances of developing heart disease in several ways. First, losing weight will directly lower your risk. Second, weight loss can help to reduce a number of risk factors for heart disease as well as lower your risk for other serious conditions. Weight loss can help to control diabetes as well as reduce high blood pressure and high blood cholesterol. Reaching a healthy weight can also help you to sleep more soundly, experience less pain from arthritis, and have more energy to take part in activities you enjoy.

Remember, if you need to lose weight, even a small weight loss will help to lower your risks of heart disease and other serious health conditions. At the very least, you should not gain any additional weight. A recent study found that young adults who maintain their weight over time, even if they are overweight, have lower risk factors for heart disease in middle age than those whose weight increases.

When it comes to weight loss, there are no quick fixes. Successful, lasting weight loss requires a change of lifestyle, not a brief effort to drop pounds quickly. Otherwise, you will probably regain the weight. Aim to lose $1/2$ pound to 2 pounds per week—no more. If you have a lot of weight to lose, ask your doctor, a registered dietitian, or a qualified nutritionist to help you develop a sensible plan for gradual weight loss.

To take off pounds and keep them off, you will need to make changes in both your eating and physical activity habits. Weight control is a question of balance. You take in calories from the food you eat. You burn off calories by physical activity. Cutting down on calories, especially calories from fat, is key to losing weight. Combining this change in diet with a regular physical activity program, such as walking or swimming, will help you both shed pounds and stay trim for the long term.

vitamins FOR HEART HEALTH

Choose Foods, Not Supplements

Until recently, it was believed that antioxidant vitamins, particularly vitamin E and beta carotene, might protect against heart disease and stroke as well as cancer. But new research shows that taking these vitamins in supplement form can be harmful—even deadly.

In the case of vitamin E supplements, a review of 19 studies showed that daily doses of 400 international units (IUs) or more may significantly increase the risk of death from all causes. Meanwhile, two major studies showed that supplementation with beta carotene (a substance that is converted to vitamin A in the liver) increases the risks of lung cancer and death in smokers. Other recent studies have shown no benefits to taking either vitamin E or beta carotene supplements to prevent cardiovascular diseases or cancer.

But studies do suggest that antioxidants in foods protect heart health. So keep eating plenty of foods that are packed with these vitamins. Foods rich in vitamin E include vegetable oils (especially safflower and sunflower oils), wheat germ, leafy green vegetables, and nuts (almonds and mixed nuts). Foods rich in beta carotene are carrots, yams, peaches, pumpkin, apricots, spinach, and broccoli.

Note: If you are taking vitamin E supplements for protection against medical conditions other than cardiovascular diseases or cancer, talk with your doctor about the risks and benefits of higher dose vitamin E supplements.

Getting Started

Anyone who has ever tried to lose weight—and keep it off—knows that it can be quite a challenge. Here are some tips to help you succeed:

Eat for health. Choose a wide variety of low-calorie, nutritious foods in moderate amounts. Include plenty of vegetables, fruits, whole grains, and low-fat or fat-free milk, as well as fish, lean meat, poultry, or dry beans. Choose foods that are low in fat and added sugars. Choose sensible portion sizes. (See "Portion Distortion" on page 91.)

Watch calories. To lose weight, most overweight people will need to cut 500 to 1,000 calories per day from their current diet. For tips on choosing low-fat, low-calorie foods, see "The Substitution Solution" on pages 92 and 93.

Keep milk on the menu. Don't cut out milk products in trying to reduce calories and fat. Milk and milk products are rich in calcium, a nutrient that helps to prevent osteoporosis, a bone-thinning disease. Instead, choose low-fat or fat-free milk products, which have the same amount of calcium as whole-milk products. Make the switch gradually. If you're used to drinking whole milk, first cut back to 2 percent, then to 1 percent, and finally to fat-free milk.

Keep moving. Physical activity is key to successful, long-term weight loss. It can help you burn calories, trim extra fat from your waist, and control your appetite. It can also tone your muscles and increase aerobic fitness. To lose weight and prevent further weight gain, gradually build up to at least 60 minutes of physical activity on most, and preferably all, days of the week. If you've already lost weight, to keep it off you'll need to get 60 to 90 minutes of daily physical activity. That may sound like a lot, but you can get results without running yourself ragged.

A recent study showed that moderate-intensity physical activity, such as brisk walking, helps people lose weight as effectively as more vigorous exercise. For more tips, see "Learn New Moves" on page 94.

Steer clear of fast food. A single meal from a fast food restaurant may pack as many calories as you need for a whole day! A recent study showed that young adults who eat frequently at fast food restaurants gain more weight and are at higher risk for diabetes in middle age than those who avoid the fast food habit. If you do eat at a fast food place, choose salads and grilled foods, and keep portion sizes small. Ask for salad dressings, mayonnaise, and other high-fat condiments to be served on the side—or not at all.

Forget the fads. Fad diets, including the high-protein, low-carbohydrate diets, are not the answer. As tempting as their promises may be, most quick-fix diets provide poor nutrition and cause many side effects, especially those with less than 800 calories per day. Although fad diets can produce fast results, most of the weight loss is due to water loss. The weight returns quickly once you stop dieting.

Know about medicines. If you are very overweight, or if you are overweight and have other weight-related risk factors or diseases, your doctor may advise you to take a medicine to help you take off pounds. You should use a weight-loss drug only after you have tried a low-calorie diet, more moderate-intensity physical activity, and other lifestyle changes for 6 months without successfully losing weight. Because weight-loss medicines have side effects, you should consider all of the risks and benefits before trying one of them. These drugs should be used along with a low-calorie eating plan and regular physical activity, not as a substitute for these lifestyle changes.

Get support. Tell your family and friends about your weight-loss plans, and let them know how they can be most helpful to you. Some women also find it useful to join a structured weight-loss program. The most effective groups provide support and advice for permanently changing eating and physical activity habits. (See "How To Choose a Weight-Loss Program" on page 89.)

Lock in your losses. After 6 months of gradually losing weight, switch your efforts to keeping the weight off by continuing to eat a nutritious, lower calorie diet and by getting 60 to 90 minutes of moderate-intensity physical activity per day. After several months of weight maintenance, talk with your health care provider about whether you need to lose additional pounds.

Seven Secrets of Successful Weight Management

If you have ever tried to take off weight, you know that it's more than a matter of promising yourself you'll eat less and move more. You also need to mentally prepare yourself for new behaviors. Here are some tips for getting and staying in a healthy weight mindset:

Start small. Many people set unrealistic goals for the amount of weight they want to lose. But you can greatly improve your health by losing just 5 to 10 percent of your starting weight. Even though you may choose to lose more weight later, keep in mind that this initial goal is both realistic and valuable.

Set smart goals. It's important to set goals that are specific, achievable, and forgiving (allow yourself to be less than perfect). For example, "exercise more" is a fine goal, but it's not very specific. "Walk for 60 minutes every day" is specific and perhaps achievable. But what if you get a bad cold one day, and there's a drenching rainstorm on another? "Walk for 60 minutes, 5 days each week" is specific, achievable, and forgiving. A great goal!

Build on success. Rather than select one big goal, choose a series of smaller goals that bring you closer and closer to your larger goal. For example, if one of your big goals is to reduce your daily calories from 2,000 to 1,200, first reduce your calories to 1,700, then move to 1,400, and finally to 1,200. Likewise, with physical activity, first establish a small new habit—such as walking 10 minutes a day—and then gradually increase it. Everyone can find time to walk 10 minutes each day. When you experience success at reaching a small goal, it will motivate you to keep moving toward your larger ones.

Reward yourself! Rewards that you control will encourage you to achieve your goals. For a reward to work well, choose something you really want, don't put off giving it to yourself, and make it dependent on meeting a specific goal. (Examples might be, "When I lose 10 pounds, I'll go to the mall the next day and get a fabulous new nail polish." or "When I've walked 60 minutes daily for 3 weeks, I'll take an afternoon off and treat myself to a movie.") Avoid food as a reward. It usually works better to give yourself frequent, small rewards for reaching short-term goals than bigger rewards that require long, difficult effort.

Write it down. Regularly record what you do on your weight-loss program, such as your daily calorie intake and amount of physical activity, as well as changes in your weight. (Try to weigh yourself at the same time of day once or twice a week.) Keeping track this way can help you and your health care provider determine what behaviors you may want to improve. Keeping tabs on your progress can also help you stay motivated.

Know your triggers. To lose weight successfully, you need to be aware of your personal eating "triggers." These are the situations that usually bring on the urge to overeat. For instance, you may get a case of the munchies while watching TV, when you see treats next to the office coffeepot, or when you're with a friend who loves to eat. To "turn off" the trigger, you'll need to make a change in the tempting situation. For example, if the pile of doughnuts near the coffeepot is hard to resist, leave the scene as soon as you pour yourself a cup of coffee.

The fine art of feeling full. Changing the way you eat can help you to eat less without feeling deprived. Eating slowly can help you feel satisfied sooner and therefore avoid second helpings. Eating lots of vegetables and fruits and drinking plenty of noncaloric beverages can also make you feel fuller. Another trick is to use smaller plates so that moderate portions don't seem skimpy. It also helps to set a regular eating schedule, especially if you tend to skip or delay meals.

How To Choose a Weight-Loss Program

Some people lose weight on their own, while others like the support of a structured program. If you decide to participate in a weight-loss program, here are some questions to ask before you join.

■ **Does the program provide counseling to help you change your eating and activity habits?**
The program should teach you how to permanently change those eating and lifestyle habits, such as lack of physical activity, that have contributed to weight gain. Research shows that people who successfully keep weight off are those who make changes in their overall lifestyles, rather than simply join a physical activity program.

■ **Does the staff include qualified health professionals, such as nutritionists, registered dietitians, doctors, nurses, psychologists, and exercise physiologists?**
Qualified professionals can help you lose weight safely and successfully. Before getting started, you'll need to be examined by a doctor if you have any health problems, currently take or plan to take any medicine, or plan to lose more than 15 to 20 pounds.

- **Does the program offer training on how to deal with times when you may feel stressed and slip back into old habits?**

  The program should provide long-term strategies for preventing and coping with possible weight problems in the future. These strategies might include setting up a support system and a regular physical activity routine.

- **Do you help make decisions on food choices and weight-loss goals?**

  In setting weight-loss goals, the program should consider your personal food likes and dislikes as well as your lifestyle. Avoid a one-strategy-fits-all program.

- **Are there fees or costs for additional items, such as dietary supplements?**

  Before you sign up, find out the total costs of participating in the program. If possible, get the costs in writing.

- **How successful is the program?**

  Few weight-loss programs gather reliable information on how well they work. Still, it is worthwhile to ask the following questions:

  - What percentage of people who start this program complete it?

  - What percentage of people experience problems or side effects? What are they?

  - What is the average weight loss among those who finish the program?

portion DISTORTION

How To Choose Sensible Servings

It's very easy to "eat with your eyes" and misjudge what equals a serving—and pile on unwanted pounds. This is especially true when you eat out, because restaurant portion sizes have been steadily expanding. Twenty years ago, the average pasta portion size was 2 cups, totaling 280 calories; today, it is 4 cups, totaling 560 calories! Use the guidelines below to keep portion sizes sensible:

- When eating out, choose small portion sizes, share an entree with a friend, or take some of the food home (if you can chill it right away).

- Check the Nutrition Facts label on product packages to learn how much food is considered a serving as well as how much fat and how many calories are in the food.

- Be especially careful to limit portion sizes of high-calorie foods, such as cookies, cakes, other sweets, sodas, french fries, oils, and spreads.

THE SUBSTITUTION SOLUTION:

Making the Switch to Low-Calorie Foods

Here are some tasty, low-calorie alternatives to old favorites. Read labels to find out how many calories are in the specific products you buy.

Instead of	Replace With
Dairy Products	
Whole milk	Low-fat or fat-free milk
Ice cream	Sorbet, sherbet, fat-free frozen yogurt, or reduced-fat ice cream
Whipping cream	Imitation whipped cream (made with fat-free milk) or low-fat vanilla yogurt
Sour cream	Plain, low-fat yogurt or fat-free sour cream
Cream cheese	Neufchâtel cheese or light or fat-free cream cheese
Cheese (sandwich types)	Reduced-calorie, low-calorie, or fat-free cheeses
Cereals and Pastas	
Ramen noodles	Brown rice or whole-grain pasta
Pasta with cheese sauce	Whole-grain pasta with red sauce or vegetables
Granola	Bran flakes, crispy rice cereals, cooked grits or oatmeal, or reduced-fat granola
Meat, Fish, Poultry	
Cold cuts, hotdogs	Low-fat cold cuts and hotdogs (watch sodium content)
Bacon or sausage	Canadian bacon or lean ham
Regular ground beef	Extra-lean ground beef or ground turkey

Instead of	Replace With
Chicken or turkey with skin	White-meat chicken or turkey without skin
Oil-packed tuna*	Water-packed tuna*
Beef (chuck, rib, brisket)	Beef (round, loin) with fat trimmed off; if possible, choose select grades
Pork (spareribs, untrimmed loin)	Pork tenderloin, trimmed; lean smoked ham loin
Whole eggs	Egg whites
Baked Goods	
Croissants, brioches, etc.	Hard French rolls or "brown 'n serve" rolls
Donuts, sweet rolls, or muffins	Reduced-fat or fat-free cookies (graham crackers, ginger snaps, fig bars)
Cake (pound, layer)	Cake (angel food, gingerbread)
Cookies	Reduced-fat or fat-free cookies (graham crackers, ginger snaps, fig bars)
Fats, Oils, Salad Dressings	
Regular margarine or butter	Light-spread, reduced-calorie, or diet margarines; look for *trans* fat-free margarines
Regular mayonnaise	Light or diet mayonnaise
Regular salad dressings	Reduced-calorie or fat-free dressings, lemon juice, or vinegars
Butter or margarine on toast	Jelly, jam, or honey on toast
Oils, shortening, or lard	Nonstick cooking spray instead of greasing pans for sauteing

*Women who are pregnant or may become pregnant, nursing mothers, and young children should avoid some types of fish and eat types lower in mercury. See the Web site www.cfsan.fda.gov/~dms/admehg3.html for more information.

Learn New Moves

Regular physical activity is a powerful way to reduce your risk of heart disease. Physical activity directly helps to prevent heart problems. Staying active also helps to prevent and control high blood pressure, keep cholesterol levels healthy, and prevent and control diabetes. Plus, regular physical activity is a great way to help take off extra pounds—and keep them off.

For women who have heart disease, regular, moderate physical activity lowers the risk of death from heart-related causes. If you have already had a heart attack, you still can benefit greatly from becoming more active. Many hospitals offer cardiac (heart) rehabilitation programs that include a wide range of physical activities. Ask your doctor for advice about the best program for you.

Regular physical activity has a host of other health benefits. It may help to prevent cancers of the breast, uterus, and colon. Staying active also strengthens the lungs, tones the muscles, keeps the joints in good condition, improves balance, and may slow bone loss. It also helps many people sleep better, feel less depressed, cope better with stress and anxiety, and generally feel more relaxed and energetic.

Women can benefit from physical activity at any age. In fact, staying active can help prevent, delay, or improve many age-related disabilities. Older women in particular may benefit from weight-bearing activities, which keep bones and muscles healthier as well as improve balance and lower the risk for serious falls. Good weight-bearing activities include carrying groceries, walking, jogging, and lifting weights. (Start with 1- to 2-pound hand weights and gradually progress to heavier weights.)

Activities that promote flexibility and balance also are important, especially for older women. Practices such as t'ai chi and yoga can improve balance and flexibility and can be done alternately with heart healthy physical activities. Check with your local recreation center, YWCA or YMCA, or adult-education program for low-cost classes in your area.

A Little Activity Goes a Long Way

The good news is that to reap benefits from physical activity, you don't have to run a marathon—or anything close to it. To reduce the risk of disease, you need only do about 30 minutes of moderate activity on most, and preferably all, days of the week. If you're trying to manage your weight and prevent gradual, unhealthy weight gain, try to boost that level to approximately 60 minutes of moderate- to vigorous-intensity physical activity on most days of the week.

Brisk walking (3 to 4 miles per hour) is an easy way to help keep your heart healthy. One study, for example, showed that regular, brisk walking reduced women's risk of heart attack by the same amount as more vigorous exercise, such as jogging. To make regular activity a pleasure rather than a chore, choose activities you enjoy. Ride a bike. Go hiking. Dance. Swim. And keep doing physical tasks around the house and yard. Trim your hedges with hand clippers. Rake leaves. Mulch your garden. Paint a room.

You can do an activity for 30 minutes at one time or choose shorter periods of at least 10 minutes each. For example, you could spend 10 minutes walking on your lunch break, another 10 minutes raking leaves in the backyard, and another 10 minutes lifting weights. The important thing is to total about 30 minutes of activity each day.

If you haven't been physically active for some time, don't let that stop you. Start slowly and gradually increase to the recommended goal. For example, if you want to begin walking regularly, begin with a 10- to 15-minute walk three times a week. As you become more fit, you can increase the number of sessions until you're doing something every day. Gradually, lengthen each walking session and quicken your pace. Before long, you will have reached your goal—walking briskly for at least 30 minutes daily to reduce the risk of disease or walking 60 minutes per day if you're also trying to manage your weight. (See "A Sample Walking Program" on page 100.)

Making Opportunities

Getting regular physical activity can be easy—especially if you take advantage of everyday opportunities to move around. For example:

- Use stairs—both up and down—instead of elevators. Start with one flight of stairs and gradually build up to more.

- Park a few blocks from the office or store and walk the rest of the way. If you take public transportation, get off a stop or two early and walk a few blocks.

- Instead of eating that rich dessert or extra snack, take a brisk stroll around the neighborhood.

- Do housework or yard work at a more vigorous pace.

- When you travel, walk around the airport, train, bus, or subway station rather than sitting and waiting.

- Keep moving while you watch TV. Lift hand weights, do some gentle yoga stretches, or pedal an exercise bike.

- Spend less time watching TV and using the computer.

- Take a movement break in the middle of the day. Get up and stretch, walk around, and give your muscles and mind a chance to relax.

Safe Moves

Some people should get medical advice before starting regular physical activity. Check with your doctor if you:

- Are over 50 years old and are not used to moderately energetic activity.

- Currently have heart trouble or have had a heart attack.

- Have a parent or sibling who developed heart disease at an early age.

- Have a chronic health problem, such as high blood pressure, diabetes, osteoporosis, or obesity.

- Tend to easily lose your balance or become dizzy.

- Feel extremely breathless after mild exertion.

- Are on any type of medication.

Once you get started, keep these guidelines in mind:

Go slow. Before each activity session, allow a 5-minute period of stretching and slow movement to give your muscles a chance to limber up and get ready for more exercise. At the end of the warmup period, gradually increase your pace. Toward the end of your activity, take another 5 minutes to cool down with a slower, less energetic pace.

Listen to your body. A certain amount of stiffness is normal at first. But if you hurt a joint or pull a muscle, stop the activity for several days to avoid more serious injury. Rest and over-the-counter painkillers properly taken can heal most minor muscle and joint problems.

Check the weather report. Dress appropriately for hot, humid days and for cold days. In all weather, drink lots of water before, during, and after physical activity.

Pay attention to warning signals. Although physical activity can strengthen your heart, some types of activity may worsen existing heart problems. Warning signals include sudden dizziness, cold sweat, paleness, fainting, or pain or pressure in your upper body just after doing a physical activity. If you notice any of these signs, call your doctor right away.

Use caution. If you're concerned about the safety of your surroundings, pair up with a buddy for outdoor activities. Walk, bike, or jog during daylight hours.

Keep at it. Unless you have to stop your activity for a health reason, stick with it. If you feel like giving up because you think you're not going as fast or as far as you should, set smaller short-term goals for yourself. If you find yourself becoming bored, try doing an activity with a friend. Or switch to another activity. The tremendous health benefits of regular, moderate-intensity physical activity are well worth the effort.

No Excuses!

We all have reasons to stay inactive. But with a little thought and planning, you can overcome most obstacles to physical activity. For example:

"I don't have time to exercise." Physical activity does take time, but remember that you can reduce your risk of disease by getting only 30 minutes of moderate-intensity activity on most days of the week. Plus, you can save time by doubling up on some activities. For example, you can ride an exercise bike or use hand weights while watching TV. Or, you can transform some of your everyday chores—like washing your car or walking the dog—into heart healthy activities by doing them more briskly than usual.

"I don't like to exercise." You may have bad memories of doing situps or running around the track in high school, forcing yourself through every sweating, panting moment. Now we know that you can get plenty of gain without pain. Activities you already do, such as gardening or walking, can improve your health. Just do more of the activities you like. Try to get friends or family members involved so that you can support each other.

"I don't have the energy to be more active." Get active first—with brief periods of moderate-intensity physical activity—and watch your energy soar. Once you begin regular physical activity, you will almost certainly feel stronger and more vigorous. As you progress, daily tasks will seem easier.

"I keep forgetting to exercise." Leave your sneakers near the door to remind yourself to walk or bring a change of clothes to work and head straight for the gym, yoga class, or walking trail on the way home. Put a note on your calendar to remind yourself to exercise. While you're at it, get in the habit of adding more activity to your daily routine.

Move It and Lose It

Activity	Calories Burned Per Hour*
Walking, 2 mph	240
Walking, 3 mph	320
Walking, 4.5 mph	440
Bicycling, 6 mph	240
Bicycling, 12 mph	410
Tennis, singles	400
Swimming, 25 yds per minute	275
Swimming, 50 yds per minute	500
Hiking	408
Cross-country skiing	700
Jumping rope	750
Jogging, 5.5 mph	740
Jogging, 7 mph	920

* For a healthy, 150-pound woman. A lighter person burns fewer calories; a heavier person burns more.

A SAMPLE WALKING PROGRAM

Warm Up	Activity	Cool Down	Total Time
Week 1 Walk slowly 5 min.	Walk briskly 5 min.	Walk slowly 5 min.	15 min.
Week 2 Walk slowly 5 min.	Walk briskly 7 min.	Walk slowly 5 min.	17 min.
Week 3 Walk slowly 5 min.	Walk briskly 9 min.	Walk slowly 5 min.	19 min.
Week 4 Walk slowly 5 min.	Walk briskly 11 min.	Walk slowly 5 min.	21 min.
Week 5 Walk slowly 5 min.	Walk briskly 13 min.	Walk slowly 5 min.	23 min.
Week 6 Walk slowly 5 min.	Walk briskly 15 min.	Walk slowly 5 min.	25 min.
Week 7 Walk slowly 5 min.	Walk briskly 18 min.	Walk slowly 5 min.	28 min.
Week 8 Walk slowly 5 min.	Walk briskly 20 min.	Walk slowly 5 min.	30 min.
Week 9 Walk slowly 5 min.	Walk briskly 23 min.	Walk slowly 5 min.	33 min.
Week 10 Walk slowly 5 min.	Walk briskly 26 min.	Walk slowly 5 min.	36 min.
Week 11 Walk slowly 5 min.	Walk briskly 28 min.	Walk slowly 5 min.	38 min.
Week 12 Walk slowly 5 min.	Walk briskly 30 min.	Walk slowly 5 min.	40 min.

You *Can* Stop Smoking

The good news is that quitting smoking immediately reduces your risk of heart disease, cancer, and other serious disorders, with the benefits increasing over time. Just 1 year after you stop smoking, your heart disease risk will drop by more than half. Within several years, it will approach the heart disease risk of someone who has never smoked. No matter how long you have been smoking, or how much, quitting will lessen your chances of developing heart disease.

If you already have heart disease, giving up cigarettes will lower your risk of a heart attack. Quitting also reduces the risk of a second heart attack in women who have already had one. There is nothing easy about giving up cigarettes. But with support and a plan of action, you *can* do it.

Getting Ready To Quit

- **Get motivated.** Take some time to think about all the benefits of being smoke free. Besides the health benefits of quitting, what else do you have to gain? Loved ones no longer exposed to secondhand smoke? A better appearance? No more standing outside in the cold or rain for a smoke? More money to spend on things besides cigarettes? Write down all of the reasons you want to stop smoking.

- **Choose a quit date.** Give yourself enough time to prepare to stop smoking—but not too much! It's best to choose a date about 2 weeks away.

- **Consider a "quit-smoking" aid.** Ask your doctor about using a medication that can help you stay off cigarettes. These aids include a patch, gum, inhaler, nasal spray, and lozenges. Some of these medicines are available over the counter. Others require a prescription. All contain very small amounts of nicotine, which can help to lessen the urge to smoke. Two other prescription quitting aids are bupropion sustained release (Zyban™), a medicine that contains no nicotine but reduces the craving for cigarettes, and varenicline tartrate (Chantix™),

"I WAS 3 MONTHS PREGNANT WITH MY SECOND CHILD WHEN I STARTED HAVING A RACING HEARTBEAT. I ENDED UP BEING DIAGNOSED WITH HYPERTROPHIC CARDIOMYOPATHY—THICKER THAN NORMAL HEART WALLS. THE CONDITION IS GENETIC, BUT I DIDN'T KNOW OF ANYONE ELSE IN MY FAMILY WHO HAD IT. I GET REGULAR CHECKUPS AND TAKE CARE OF MY OVERALL HEALTH, AND I TEACH MY KIDS TO MAINTAIN A HEALTHY LIFESTYLE. MY DAUGHTERS HAVE BEEN SCREENED FOR HEART DISEASE."

—Shannon

which both eases withdrawal symptoms and blocks the effects of nicotine if you slip and begin smoking again. If you decide to use one of these medicines, be sure to talk with your doctor about how to use it properly.

- **Line up support.** Many women find that quitting smoking is easier with the support of others. Tell your family, friends, and coworkers that you plan to quit and let them know how they can help you. For example, if someone close to you smokes, ask him or her not to smoke around you. (It is easier to quit when people around you aren't smoking.) You might also find a support group or Internet chat room helpful. Plan to get in touch with your "support team" regularly to share your progress and to get encouragement. If possible, quit with a friend or family member.

- **Make a fresh start.** The day before you quit, get rid of all cigarettes in your home, your car, or at work. (Keeping a few cigarettes "just in case I need them" will lower your chances of success.) Throw away ashtrays, matches, and lighters. Many women like to quit with a clean, fresh home or car that is free of cigarette odor. You may want to clean the drapes or shampoo the carpet of your home or car. After quitting, you'll enjoy the new scents as your sense of smell returns.

Breaking the Habit

- **Know what to expect.** The first few weeks can be tough. Most people experience strong urges to smoke as well as withdrawal symptoms, such as headaches, difficulty sleeping, trouble concentrating, and feeling cranky or nervous. While these reactions are not pleasant, it's important to know that they are signs that your body is recovering from smoking. Within a few weeks, most people already feel much better.

- **Know yourself.** To quit successfully, you need to know your personal smoking "triggers." These are the situations and feelings that usually bring on the urge to light up. Some common triggers are drinking coffee, having an alcoholic drink, talking on the phone, watching someone else smoke, and experiencing stress or depression. Make a list of your own personal triggers and avoid as many of them as you can. For those you can't avoid, plan now for how you will deal with them.

- **Find new habits.** Replace your triggers with new activities that you don't associate with smoking. For example, if you have always had a cigarette with a cup of coffee, switch to tea for a while. If stress is a trigger for you, try a relaxation exercise such as deep breathing to calm yourself. (Take a slow, deep breath, count to five, and release it. Repeat 10 times.)

- **Keep busy.** Get involved in activities that require you to use your hands, such as needlework, jigsaw puzzles, or fixup projects around your house or apartment. When you feel the urge to put something in your mouth, try some vegetable sticks, apple slices, or sugarless gum. Some people find it helpful to inhale on a straw or chew on a toothpick until the urge passes.

- **Keep moving.** Walk, garden, bike, or do some yoga stretches. Physical activity will make you feel better and help prevent weight gain.

- **Be good to yourself.** Get plenty of rest, drink lots of water, and eat three healthy meals each day. If you are not as productive or cheerful as usual during the first weeks after quitting, be gentle with yourself. Give yourself a chance to adjust to being a nonsmoker. Congratulate yourself for making a major, positive change in your life.

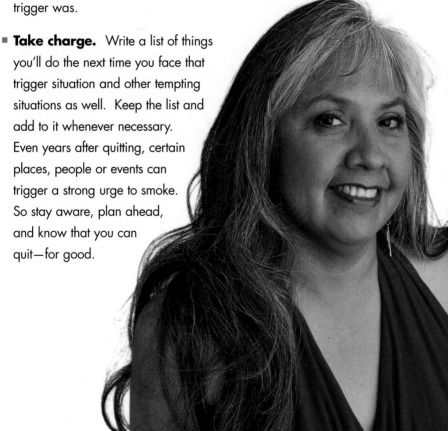

If You Slip

A slip means that you've had a small setback and smoked a cigarette after your quit date. This is most likely to happen during the first 3 months after quitting. Below are three suggestions to help you get right back on the nonsmoking track:

- **Don't be discouraged.** Having a cigarette or two doesn't mean you can't quit smoking. A slip happens to many, many people who successfully quit. Keep thinking of yourself as a nonsmoker. You are one.

- **Learn from experience.** What was the trigger that made you light up? Were you driving home from work, having a glass of wine at a party, or feeling angry with your boss? Think back on the day's events until you remember what the trigger was.

- **Take charge.** Write a list of things you'll do the next time you face that trigger situation and other tempting situations as well. Keep the list and add to it whenever necessary. Even years after quitting, certain places, people or events can trigger a strong urge to smoke. So stay aware, plan ahead, and know that you can quit—for good.

five AIDS FOR QUITTING

As you prepare to quit smoking, consider using a medication that can help you stay off cigarettes. Some of these medications contain very small amounts of nicotine, which can help to lessen the urge to smoke. They include nicotine gum (available over the counter), the nicotine patch (available over the counter and by prescription), a nicotine inhaler (by prescription only), and a nicotine nasal spray (by prescription only). Another quitting aid is bupropion sustained release (Zyban™), a medicine that contains no nicotine but reduces the craving for cigarettes. Varenicline tartrate (Chantix™) eases withdrawl symptoms and blocks the effects of nicotine if you slip and start smoking again. Both are available only by prescription. While all of these medications can help people to stop smoking, they are not safe for everyone. Talk with your doctor about whether you should try any of these aids.

A WEIGHTY *concern*

Many women fear that if they stop smoking, they will gain unwanted weight. But most exsmokers gain less than 10 pounds. Weight gain may be partly due to changes in the way the body uses calories after smoking stops. Some people also may gain weight because they substitute high-calorie food for cigarettes. Choosing lower calorie foods and getting more physical activity can reduce the amount of weight you gain.

If you do put on some weight, you can work on losing it after you have become comfortable as a nonsmoker. Meanwhile, concentrate on becoming smoke free—your heart health depends on it.

FOR WOMEN *who* HAVE HEART DISEASE

*I*f you have heart disease, it is extremely important to control it. Eating well, engaging in regular physical activity, and maintaining a healthy weight will help to lessen the severity of your condition. If you smoke, you'll need to quit. And if you have diabetes, you will need to manage it carefully.

You also may need certain tests, medications, or special procedures. This section explains each of these and how they can help to protect your heart health.

Screening Tests

In most cases, you will need some tests to find out for sure if you have heart disease and how severe it is. If your doctor doesn't mention tests, be sure to ask whether they could be helpful. Most screening tests are done outside the body and are painless. After taking a careful medical history and doing a physical examination, your doctor may give you one or more of the following tests:

- **Electrocardiogram** (ECG or EKG) makes a graph of the heart's electrical activity as it beats. This test can show abnormal heartbeats, heart muscle damage, blood flow problems in the coronary arteries, and heart enlargement.

- **Stress test** (or treadmill test or exercise ECG) records the heart's electrical activity during exercise, usually on a treadmill or exercise bike. The test can detect whether the heart is getting enough blood and oxygen. If you are unable to exercise due to arthritis or another health condition, a stress test can be done without exercise. Instead, you will be given a medicine that increases blood flow to the heart muscle and makes the heart beat faster, mimicking the changes that occur when you exercise. This test is usually followed by a nuclear scan or echocardiography to see whether there are any problems with the blood flow to the heart.

- **Nuclear scan** shows the working of the heart muscle as blood flows through the heart. A small amount of radioactive material is injected into a vein, usually in the arm, and a camera records how much is taken up by the heart muscle.

- **Echocardiography** changes sound waves into pictures that show the heart's size, shape, and movement. The sound waves are also used to see how much blood is pumped out by the heart when it contracts.

- **Cardiac catheterization** is a medical procedure used to diagnose and treat certain heart conditions. A long, thin, flexible tube called a catheter is put into a blood vessel in the arm or upper thigh (groin) and threaded up into the heart. Through the catheter, the doctor can perform diagnostic tests and treatments on the heart. The diagnostic tests include the following:

  - *Coronary angiography* (or angiogram or arteriography) shows an x ray of blood flow problems and blockages in the coronary arteries. A dye is injected into the catheter, allowing the heart and blood vessels to be filmed as the heart pumps. The picture is called an angiogram or arteriogram.

  - *Ventriculogram* is sometimes a part of the x-ray dye test described above. It is used to get a picture of the heart's main pumping chamber, typically the left ventricle.

  - *Intracoronary ultrasound* may be done during a cardiac catheterization to measure blood flow. It gives a picture of the coronary arteries that shows the thickness and other features of the artery wall. This lets the doctor see blood flow and any blockages.

COULD YOU HAVE *hidden* HEART DISEASE?

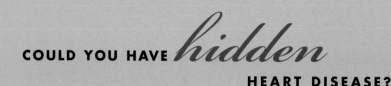

Many women have undiagnosed heart disease—even after getting tested for it. New research shows that up to 3 million women in the United States have a hard-to-spot form of heart disease called "coronary microvascular syndrome," in which plaque spreads evenly throughout the walls of very small arteries, rather than building up in a larger, main artery. Even though women with this condition have insufficient blood and oxygen flow to the heart muscle, a standard angiogram (which is designed to pick up blockages in large arteries) is likely to show their arteries to be normal.

This means that women with heart disease symptoms should be prepared to speak up to their doctors. If you receive a "normal" angiogram but still have chest pain or other heart symptoms, ask your doctor whether you might have a problem with the functioning of your small arteries. To find out, you may be asked to undergo relatively simple tests, such as a questionnaire that measures how easily you can perform everyday tasks. This quiz, called the "Duke Activity Status Index," can help to predict your heart attack risk.

In addition, several new, highly sensitive screening tests have been developed. Ask your doctor about these tests:

- **Carotid doppler ultrasound** uses sound waves to detect blockages and narrowing of the carotid artery in the neck. Both conditions can signal an increased risk for heart attack or stroke.

- **Electron-beam computed tomography (EBCT)** is a super fast scan that provides a snapshot of the calcium buildup in your coronary arteries. It may predict whether you'll be at higher risk for heart disease in the future. This test is promising, but not foolproof, and requires careful evaluation by your doctor.

- **Magnetic resonance imaging (MRI)** is a scan using magnets and computers to create high-quality images of the heart's structure and functioning. It is often used to evaluate congenital heart disease. The test can also detect severe blockages in coronary arteries in people who are having unstable angina or a heart attack, thereby allowing immediate treatment to restore blood flow to the heart.

aspirin: TAKE WITH CAUTION

This well-known "wonder drug" can help to lower the risk of a heart attack or stroke for those who have already had one. It can also help to keep arteries open in those who have had a previous heart bypass or other artery-opening procedure, such as angioplasty. In addition, aspirin is given to people who arrive at a hospital emergency department with a suspected heart attack or stroke.

It's important to know that aspirin has not been approved by the U.S. Food and Drug Administration for the prevention of heart attacks in those who have never had a heart attack or stroke.

However, a recent large study has found that among healthy women, taking low-dose aspirin every other day may help to prevent a first stroke. Among women over the age of 65, low-dose aspirin every other day may also prevent a first heart attack. If you are considering taking aspirin for this purpose, keep in mind that it is a powerful drug with many side effects. It can also mix dangerously with other drugs, including some over-the-counter medicines and dietary supplements.

If you're thinking about using aspirin either to treat or prevent heart problems, talk with your doctor first. Only a doctor who knows your medical history and current health condition can judge whether the benefits would outweigh the risks. If aspirin is a good choice for you, be sure to take the dose recommended by your doctor.

If your doctor does advise you to take aspirin, be sure to continue practicing the "Big Four" heart healthy habits—eating nutritiously, getting regular physical activity, maintaining a healthy weight, and for those who smoke, quitting. Aspirin can be a useful treatment for some people, but it is not a substitute for a healthy lifestyle.

Medications

To control or prevent heart disease, you may need to take medicine. Medications may be used to treat a risk factor, such as high blood pressure or high blood cholesterol, or relieve the chest pain that often accompanies heart disease. If you do take medicine, it's important to keep up your heart healthy lifestyle, because healthy daily habits will keep your dose of medicine as low as possible. Medications that are commonly prescribed for people with heart disease include the following:

- **ACE (angiotensin converting enzyme) inhibitors** stop the body from producing a chemical that narrows blood vessels. They are used to treat high blood pressure and damaged heart muscle. ACE inhibitors may reduce the risks of a future heart attack and heart failure. They also can prevent kidney damage in some people with diabetes.

- **Anticoagulants** decrease the ability of the blood to clot, and therefore help to prevent clots from forming in your arteries and blocking blood flow. (These medicines are sometimes called "blood thinners," though they do not actually thin the blood.) Anticoagulants will not dissolve clots that have already formed, but these medicines may prevent the clots from becoming larger and causing more serious problems.

- **Antiplatelets** are medications that stop blood particles called platelets from clumping together to form harmful clots. These medications may be given to people who have had a heart attack, who have angina, or who experience chest pain after an angioplasty procedure. Aspirin is one type of antiplatelet medicine. (See "Aspirin: Take With Caution," on page 111.)

- **Beta blockers** slow the heart and allow it to beat with less force. They are used to treat high blood pressure and some arrhythmias (abnormal heart rhythms) and to prevent a repeat heart attack. They can also delay or prevent the development of angina.

- **Calcium-channel blockers** relax blood vessels. They are used to treat high blood pressure, angina, and some arrhythmias.

- **Digitalis** makes the heart contract harder and is used when the heart can't pump strongly enough on its own. It also slows down some fast heart rhythms.

- **Diuretics** (water pills) decrease fluid in the body and are very effective in treating high blood pressure. New research suggests that diuretics also can help to prevent stroke, heart attack, and heart failure. For those who already have heart failure, diuretics can help to reduce fluid buildup in the lungs and swelling in the feet and ankles.

- **Nitrates** relax blood vessels and relieve chest pain. Nitrates in different forms can be used to relieve the pain of an angina attack, to prevent an expected episode, or to reduce the number of attacks that occur by using the medicine regularly on a long-term basis. The most commonly used nitrate for angina is nitroglycerin.

- **Menopausal hormone therapy** was once thought to lower the risk of heart attack and stroke for women with heart disease. But research now shows that women with heart disease should not take it. Menopausal hormone therapy can involve the use of estrogen alone or estrogen plus progestin. For women with heart disease, estrogen alone will not prevent heart attacks, and estrogen plus progestin increases the risk for heart attack during the first few years of use. Estrogen plus progestin also increases the risk for blood clots, stroke, and breast cancer.

Special Procedures

Advanced heart disease may require special procedures to open an artery and improve blood flow. These operations are usually done to ease severe chest pain or clear blood vessel blockages. They include the following:

- **Coronary angioplasty, or balloon angioplasty.** In this procedure, a thin tube called a catheter is threaded through an artery into the heart's narrowed blood vessel. The catheter has a tiny balloon at its tip, which is repeatedly inflated and deflated to open and stretch the artery, improving blood flow. Often, a tiny tube called a stent is permanently inserted in the artery to keep it open. Stenting may be particularly beneficial for women.

- **Coronary artery bypass graft, or "bypass surgery."** A piece of vein is taken from the leg or a section of an artery is taken from the chest or wrist. This piece is attached to the heart artery both above and below the narrowed area, making a bypass around the blockage. If you need bypass surgery, ask your doctor whether you are a candidate for one of the newer types of bypass procedures. Inquire about "off pump" and "minimally invasive" coronary bypass surgery.

GETTING HELP FOR A *heart* ATTACK

For many people, the first symptom of heart disease is a heart attack. Therefore, every woman should know how to identify the symptoms of a heart attack and how to get immediate medical help. Ideally, treatment should start within 1 hour of the first symptoms. Recognizing the warning signs and getting help quickly can save your life.

Know the Warning Signs

Not all heart attacks begin with sudden, crushing pain, as is often shown on TV or in the movies. Many heart attacks start slowly as mild pain or discomfort. The most common warning signs for women and men are listed below:

- **Chest discomfort.** Most heart attacks involve discomfort in the center of the chest that lasts more than a few minutes. It may feel like uncomfortable pressure, squeezing, fullness, or pain. The discomfort can be mild or severe, and it may come and go.

- **Discomfort in other areas of the upper body,** including one or both arms, the back, neck, jaw, or stomach.

- **Shortness of breath.** This symptom may occur along with or without chest discomfort.

- **Other signs** include nausea, light-headedness, or breaking out in a cold sweat.

Get Help Quickly

If you think you, or someone else, may be having a heart attack, you must act quickly to prevent disability or death. Wait no more than a few minutes—5 minutes at most—before dialing 9–1–1.

It is important to dial 9–1–1 because emergency medical personnel can begin treatment even before you get to the hospital. They also have the equipment and training to start your heart beating again if it stops. Dialing 9–1–1 quickly can save your life.

Even if you're not sure you're having a heart attack, dial 9–1–1 if your symptoms last up to 5 minutes. If your symptoms stop completely in less than 5 minutes, you should still call your doctor.

You also must act at once because hospitals have clot-busting medicines and other artery-opening treatments and procedures that can stop a heart attack, if given quickly. These treatments work best when given within the first hour after a heart attack starts.

Women tend to delay longer than men in getting help for a possible heart attack. A large study of heart attack patients found that, on average, women waited 22 minutes longer than men did before going to the hospital. Many women delay because they don't want to bother or worry others, especially if their symptoms turn out to be a false alarm. But when you're facing something as serious as a possible heart attack, it is much better to be safe than sorry. If you have any symptoms of a possible heart attack that last up to 5 minutes, call 9–1–1 right away.

When you get to the hospital, don't be afraid to speak up for what you need—or bring someone who can speak up for you. Ask for tests that can determine if you are having a heart attack. Commonly given initial tests include an electrocardiogram (ECG or EKG) and a cardiac enzyme blood test (to check for heart damage).

At the hospital, don't let anyone tell you that your symptoms are "just indigestion" or that you're "overreacting." You have the right to be thoroughly examined for a possible heart attack. If you are having a heart attack, you have the right to immediate treatment to help stop the attack.

Plan Ahead

Nobody plans on having a heart attack. But just as many people have a plan in case of fire, it is important to develop a plan to deal with a possible heart attack. Taking the following steps can preserve your health—and your life:

- Learn the heart attack warning signs by heart.

- Talk with family and friends about the warning signs and the need to call 9–1–1 quickly.

- Talk with your health care provider about your risk factors for heart attack and how to reduce them.

- Write out a heart attack survival plan that has vital medical information and keep it handy. (Use the accompanying box on page 118 as a guide.)

- Arrange in advance to have someone care for your children or other dependents in an emergency.

If you think you, or someone else, may be having a heart attack, you must act quickly to prevent disability or death. Wait no more than a few minutes—5 at most—before dialing 9-1-1.

HEART ATTACK *survival* PLAN

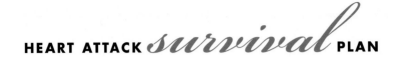

Fill out the form below and make several copies of it. Keep one copy near your home phone, another at work, and a third copy in your wallet or purse.

Information To Share With Emergency Medical Personnel and Hospital Staff

Medicines you are taking: _____

_____

_____

Medicines you are allergic to: _____

_____

_____

How To Contact Your Doctor

If symptoms stop completely in less than 5 minutes, you should still call your doctor right away.

Phone number during office hours: _____

Phone number after office hours: _____

Person To Contact If You Go to the Hospital

Name: _____

Home phone number: _____

Work phone number: _____

Cell phone number: _____

THE HEART OF THE *matter*

Getting serious about heart health may seem like a huge project. Because it means making changes in daily living habits, for many women it is a major effort. But it doesn't have to be an overwhelming one. Some people find it easier to tackle only one habit at a time. For example, if you smoke cigarettes and also eat a diet high in saturated fats, work on quitting smoking first. Then, once you've become used to life without cigarettes, begin to skim the fat from your diet.

And remember, nobody's perfect. Nobody always eats the ideal diet or gets just the right amount of physical activity. Few smokers are able to swear off cigarettes without a slip or two along the way. The important thing is to follow a sensible, realistic plan that will gradually lessen your chances of developing heart disease or help you to control it.

Women are taking a more active role in their own health care. We are asking more questions, and we are readier than ever to make changes that will help us lead healthier lives. We are concerned not only about treatment, but also about the prevention of many disorders that commonly strike women. Taking steps to prevent and control heart disease is part of this growing movement to take charge of our own health. The reward of a healthy heart—a better chance for a longer, more vigorous life—is well worth the effort.

HOW TO ESTIMATE YOUR *risk*

*U*se these risk tables to find your chances of having a heart attack in the next 10 years, given as a percentage. (For more on this, see page 59.)

	Points		Points
Age 20–34	-7	Age 55–59	8
Age 35–39	-3	Age 60–64	10
Age 40–44	0	Age 65–69	12
Age 45–49	3	Age 70–74	14
Age 50–54	6	Age 75–79	16

	Points				
Total Cholesterol	Age 20-39	Age 40-49	Age 50-59	Age 60-69	Age 70-79
<160	0	0	0	0	0
160–199	4	3	2	1	1
200–239	8	6	4	2	1
240–279	11	8	5	3	2
≥280	13	10	7	4	2

	Points				
	Age 20-39	Age 40-49	Age 50-59	Age 60-69	Age 70-79
Nonsmoker	0	0	0	0	0
Smoker	9	7	4	2	1

HDL (mg/dL)	Points	HDL (mg/dL)	Points
60	-1	40–49	1
50–59	0	<40	2

	Points			Points	
Systolic BP (mmHg)	If Untreated	If Treated	Systolic BP (mmHg)	If Untreated	If Treated
<120	0	0	140–159	3	5
120–129	1	3	≥160	4	6
130–139	2	4			

Point Total	10-Year Risk %	Point Total	10-Year Risk %	Point Total	10-Year Risk %
<9	<1	14	2	20	11
9	1	15	3	21	14
10	1	16	4	22	17
11	1	17	5	23	22
12	1	18	6	24	27
13	2	19	8	25	30

(Framingham Heart Study Point Scores)

TO *learn* MORE

To find out more about preventing and controlling heart disease, contact the following information sources:

NHLBI Health Information Center
P.O. Box 30105
Bethesda, MD 20824-0105
Phone: 301-592-8573
TTY: 240-629-3255
Fax: 301-592-8563

Provides information on the prevention and treatment of heart disease and offers publications on heart disease and heart health.

Also, check out these NHLBI heart health Web sites and Web pages:

■ NHLBI Web site: **www.nhlbi.nih.gov**

■ Diseases and Conditions A–Z Index: **www.nhlbi.nih.gov/health/dci/index.html**

■ *The Heart Truth*: A National Awareness Campaign for Women About Heart Disease: **www.hearttruth.gov**

■ NHLBI "Your Guide To Better Health" Series: **http://hp2010.nhlbihin.net/yourguide**
  • "Your Guide to a Healthy Heart"
  • "Your Guide to Living Well With Heart Disease"
  • "Your Guide to Lowering Your Blood Pressure With DASH"
  • "Your Guide to Lowering Your Cholesterol With TLC"
  • "Your Guide to Physical Activity and Your Heart"
  • "Your Guide to Healthy Sleep"

■ "Keep the Beat: Heart Healthy Recipes from the NHLBI": **www.nhlbi.nih.gov/health/public/heart/other/ktb_recipebk/**

Interactive Web Pages

■ Your Guide to Lowering High Blood Pressure: **www.nhlbi.nih.gov/hbp/index.html**

■ Live Healthier, Live Longer (on lowering elevated blood cholesterol): **www.nhlbi.nih.gov/chd**

■ High Blood Cholesterol: What You Need To Know: **www.nhlbi.nih.gov/health/public/heart/chol/hbc_what.htm**

- Aim for a Healthy Weight:
  www.nhlbi.nih.gov/health/public/heart/obesity/lose_wt/index.htm

- Act in Time to Heart Attack Signs:
  www.nhlbi.nih.gov/actintime/index.htm

- We Can! (Ways to Enhance Children's Activity and Nutrition):
  http://wecan.nhlbi.nih.gov

- Stay in Circulation: Take Steps to Learn About P.A.D.:
  www.aboutpad.org

Additional Resources

- National Diabetes Information Clearinghouse:
  http://diabetes.niddk.nih.gov

- Help for Quitting Smoking:
  www.cancer.gov/cancertopics/factsheet/Tobacco

- American Heart Association: **www.americanheart.org**

- Heart Healthy Women: **www.hearthealthywomen.org**

- National Women's Health Information Center, Office on Women's Health, U.S. Department of Health and Human Services: **www.womenshealth.gov**

- WomenHeart: the National Coalition for Women with Heart Disease:
  www.womenheart.org

- For still more information on heart health, see MedlinePlus:
  http://medlineplus.gov/